All rights reserved. Copyright Natalie Duhon 2022.

User may reproduce this document for use in immediate family only. Do not share this document with anyone outside of your immediate family. Licensed clinicians may reproduce this document to use with their caseload. Teachers may reproduce this document for use in their classroom. All other copies of this document are unauthorized without expressed and written consent. This includes, but is not limited to, the document being transmitted by electronic reproduction.

This resource is intended for informational purposes only. It is not intended to be used as a diagnostic tool or a replacement for treatment or medical intervention. Mental health/medical emergencies should be addressed immediately with a licensed provider in your area.

Scripture taken from the International Children's Bible®. Copyright © 1986, 1988, 1999 by Thomas Nelson. Used by permission. All rights reserved.

Cover image and feelings faces by: © Lauren Sibley Brasseaux

All other images purchased through Creative Market and are licensed for commercial use.

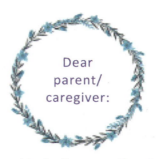

Dear parent/caregiver:

Anger frustration, confusion, and sadness…big feelings manifest in many ways. Many of us may not have been taught how to identify and manage our emotions as young children. We may have been told "big boys don't cry" or "ladies can't get angry." The reality is we experience emotions because God made us to be human. We can learn to express them in a healthy way. Stuffing our emotions can lead to many issues, including physical ones such as upset stomach, muscle tension, or headaches. More life threatening issues include suicidal thoughts/attempts, self-harm, and addictive behavior. This resource is designed to help educate you, the parent/caregiver, as you begin to educate your child. This resource is designed for you and your child to use together.

Some lessons will have a "for parent/caregiver" section. (These will be in purple text so they are easy to identify). It is up to you whether or not you feel your child is mature enough to read it. This book is not intended to just be handed over to your child to read as it contains information that your child may not be ready to handle just yet. I've also included parent/caregiver journal prompts to help you on your journey. This book does not need to be read in a particular order. Feel free to choose the lessons that are most needed in your family, but always read the parent/caregiver information first. Since this book is designed for elementary, some activities may seem too mature for a Kindergartener or first grader. That's okay! Use what works for you now and save the rest for a later date. I highly encourage you, the parent/caregiver, to try therapy for yourself. It can be a life changing experience and beneficial even if you are not in crisis.

The information in this book is based on my ten plus years of experience in the mental health field. Several resources have been consulted to ensure the information in this book is accurate and follows evidenced based practice. Several colleagues have been consulted as well. I have listed my most commonly consulted resources in the references list at the end of this book. I am also required to complete forty continuing education hours every two years, on a variety of topics related to mental health. Research in mental health is continuously advancing and the information in this book is as up to date as possible at the time of publication. I contemplated adding the topic of grief, but ultimately decided against it due to the complex and sensitive nature of it. In-person counseling with a licensed therapist, play therapist, or pastor is highly recommended when a child is experiencing grief.

This resource is intended for informational purposes only. It is not intended as a diagnostic tool or treatment. If you need further help or suspect your child is in danger, please seek medical help immediately. If a child is experiencing difficulty functioning in their daily activities, it is recommended you seek professional help. Mental health professionals all over the country and world are ready to assist you and your child further if needed. These include psychiatrists, psychiatric nurse practitioners, licensed counselors, licensed social workers, and psychologists. Your local pediatrician or general practitioner can help point you in the direction of resources in your area. There are also helpful resources listed in the back of this book.

"Tell the greatness of the Lord with me.
Let us praise his name together.
I asked the Lord for help, and he answered me.
He saved me from all that I feared.
Those who go to Him for help are happy.
They are never disgraced."
Psalm 34:3-5 (International Children's Bible)

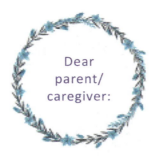

Dear parent/caregiver:

How would you define the word emotion? One way to describe our emotions is how we feel. Words we frequently use include happy, sad, mad, and worried. There are many ways to describe our emotions and many ways to manage them. Some of these are helpful, but there are many things we tend to do that are unhelpful. If we don't manage our emotions, we can suffer severe consequences. These might include negative thoughts, physical issues, and poor behavior.

Webster's dictionary (2022) defines emotion as "a conscious mental reaction (such as anger or fear) subjectively experienced as strong feeling usually directed toward a specific object and typically accompanied by physiological and behavioral changes in the body."

As parents/caregivers, it is our job and our privilege to help our children learn to identify and manage their emotions in a healthy way. As always, looking to the Bible as our primary source can help us teach them (and ourselves) healthy ways to express ourselves in ways that honor God.

Throughout this curriculum, I will reference the Bible as well as recommend hymns. You can read, listen to, or journal about them.

Just like medication is sometimes needed for a person with diabetes or other physical issues, medication is sometimes necessary to address issues with mental health. Please consult with a mental health provider in your area.

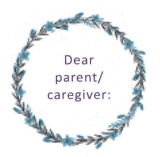

Dear parent/caregiver:

Journaling is an incredibly helpful skill that has been researched extensively to demonstrate its effectiveness. I will recommend journaling opportunities throughout this book, both for you and your child. If your child is unable to read/write fluently, they can dictate their journal to you or draw pictures. (You may also prefer to draw pictures. Choose what works for you!) Writing down and memorizing Bible verses that apply to your unique situation can also be beneficial.

I challenge you, as a parent/caregiver, to think about your own mental health before beginning this book with your child. I encourage you to keep your own journal during this experience, beginning with some of these questions.

Growing up, what did you learn about emotions? What were you taught or NOT taught? Did your parents teach you about emotions or did you learn by what you observed? These can be explicit or implicit lessons about how to think and feel. What were the most common emotions expressed by your parents? Siblings? Other caregivers? Is there a common theme that was expressed in your family? Was it more positive or more negative?

As an adult, how do you manage your emotions? What role does your faith play in how you manage difficult emotions? What's the theme in your home? (stressed, angry, peaceful, etc.) What do you want it to be? What do you do well and what do you want to improve?

What significant events in your life have shaped you as an individual, a spouse, and a parent?

Have you ever been to therapy for your own growth? Have you ever spoken to your pastor about issues you've faced?

How have you coped with stress in the past? (Healthy and unhealthy ways)

*Your journal is not meant to be shared with your children. However, I encourage you to share it with your spouse, therapist, or pastor.

Your child will be frequently prompted to either discuss or journal during this curriculum. I highly recommend older children having their own journal. Younger children who have limited writing skills may find it helpful to draw what they're learning. These activities, along with good discussion and narration, will help ensure your child is learning the information well.

*Narration is a skill that is often utilized in a Charlotte Mason education. It involves a student retelling what was just read to demonstrate understanding. There are many resources and videos that explain this technique in depth. Although it is not a counseling skill, it is very helpful in learning and retaining information.

Table of Contents

Chapter 1: Introduction to Emotions
Chapter 2: Anger
Chapter 3: Anxiety
Chapter 4: Relaxation
Chapter 5: Sadness
Chapter 6: Happiness, Peace, and Gratitude
Chapter 7: Self-esteem
Chapter 8: Self-care
Chapter 9: Love
Chapter 10: Social and Communication Skills
Chapter 11: Conflict
Chapter 12: Boundaries
Chapter 13: Forgiveness
Chapter 14: Support System
Chapter 15: Habits and Goals
Chapter 16: Automatic Thoughts
Chapter 17: Problem-solving
Chapter 18: Coping Skills
Chapter 19: Biblical Learning to Improve Mental Health
Chapter 20: Learning From Real Life Situations
Appendix

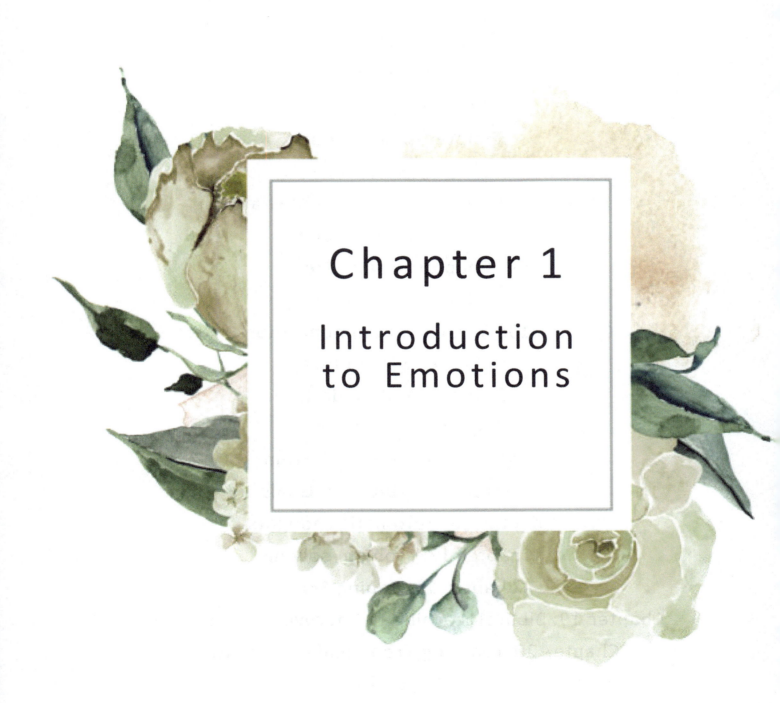

Chapter 1
Introduction to Emotions

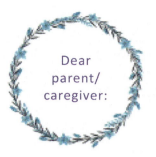

Dear parent/caregiver:

Emotions help us experience life more fully. However, they can also cause us significant distress if not managed appropriately. Recognizing and listening to our emotions can let us know when our needs are not being met and when we need to ask for help.

It's important to remember that God created us with a purpose. Our emotions have a specific purpose too! They can motivate us, alert us that we need something, or help us understand ourselves better. Fear motivates us to take steps to ensure we are safe. If I see a stray dog, I will be cautious before approaching it because I know it may be dangerous. Anger can motivate us to ensure we and our loved ones are safe and our needs are being met. If I feel like my loved ones are being treated unfairly, anger will motivate me to advocate for them. Love motivates us to care for ourselves and others. Sadness can alert us to unmet needs or expectations.

This book aims to help understand how to become more aware of emotions and healthy ways to manage them. The more we understand ourselves, the more we will be able to understand others.

As you work through this curriculum, take the time to point out to your child emotions you see in daily life. This can include movies, books, and daily life at home. Use descriptive words to help them see what that emotion looks like.

Example: "Did you see the little girl on the show? She frowned and put her head down. Now her arms are crossed and she doesn't want to talk to anyone. How do you think she's feeling? What happened that might have caused her to feel this way?" (Feeling words may include: sad, lonely, jealous, unhappy, etc.). Picture books are another great way to learn about emotions, especially the ones with detailed illustrations. Be on the lookout for how emotions are depicted in what you are already using at home!

Draw a face to describe each emotion. What is happening in your life when you experience these emotions? Don't forget to share with a loved one! Do you know any other emotion words? If you don't, that's okay! We'll be learning about lots of emotion words in this book.

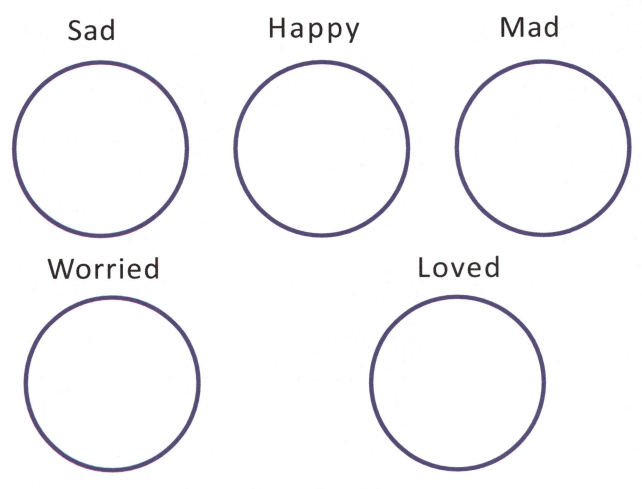

Draw how you feel here:

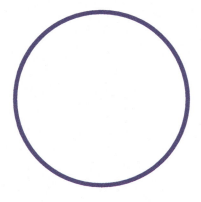

Emotions list

Take some time reading through these words and discussing the ones you and your child know. Circle the ones you don't know. We will learn more about these throughout this curriculum.

angry	loving	delighted
mad	nervous	apprehensive
sad	happy	glad
lonely	disappointed	inspired
ashamed	embarrassed	peaceful
scared	joyful	relaxed
worried	stressed	merry
anxious	fearful	ecstatic
depressed	annoyed	proud
upset	exasperated	surprised
uneasy	brave	antsy
calm	confident	furious
bored	cheerful	panicked
determined	bitter	grateful
guilty	sorrowful	appreciated
frustrated	unloved	forlorn
frightened	content	gloomy
jealous	loved	hopeful
confused	irritated	excited

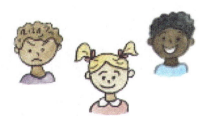

© Natalie Duhon

Write as many words as you can to describe your emotions. Then use your emotion cards to play a game of memory match! When you get a pair, talk about something that helps you feel better or something that helps you feel happy! (This is a game that you can play throughout this curriculum as you and your child become more comfortable learning about and expressing emotions).

Another activity you can do is have your child pick an emotion card. Then, write a few sentences that tell a story about why the child feels that way.

_____

_____

_____

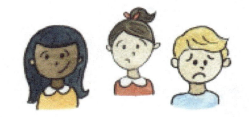

Emotions guessing game: Pick an emotion card. You have one minute to have your partner guess what you are feeling…without using words! Then switch. Talk about how much our body language shows how we're feeling, even when we don't use words! (Examples of body language include: crossed arms, nodding our head, shrugging our shoulders, smiling or frowning, etc.). These will be further addressed in the lesson on communication skills. I recommend you do this exercise several times throughout this curriculum.

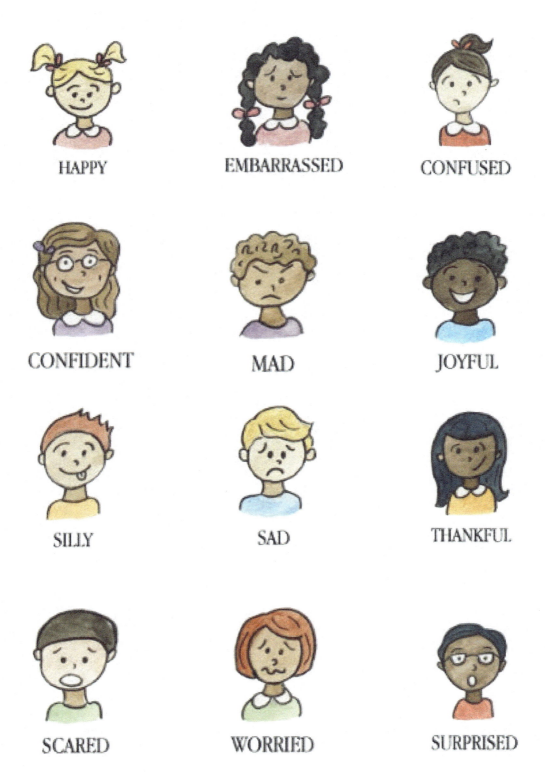

Intentionally left blank for double sided printing

Emotion cards (I recommend you laminate these. You will be directed to use them for various activities throughout the curriculum.)

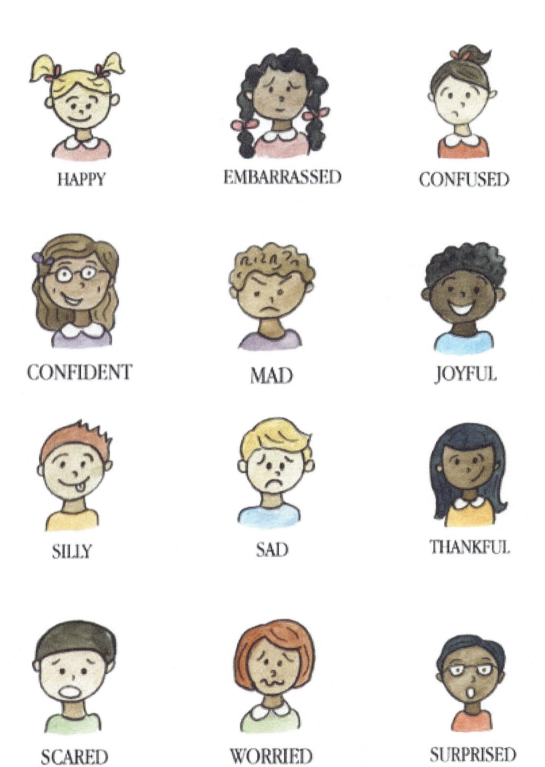

Intentionally left blank for double sided printing

Emotion cards

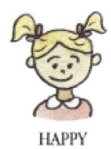 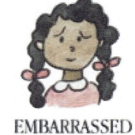 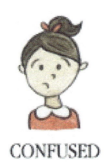

HAPPY   EMBARRASSED   CONFUSED

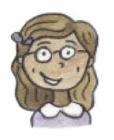 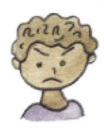 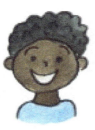

CONFIDENT   MAD   JOYFUL

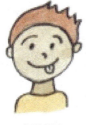 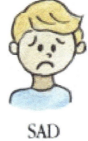 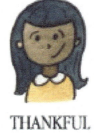

SILLY   SAD   THANKFUL

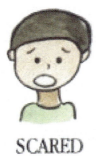 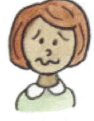 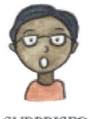

SCARED   WORRIED   SURPRISED

Intentionally left blank for double sided printing

Junto wheel

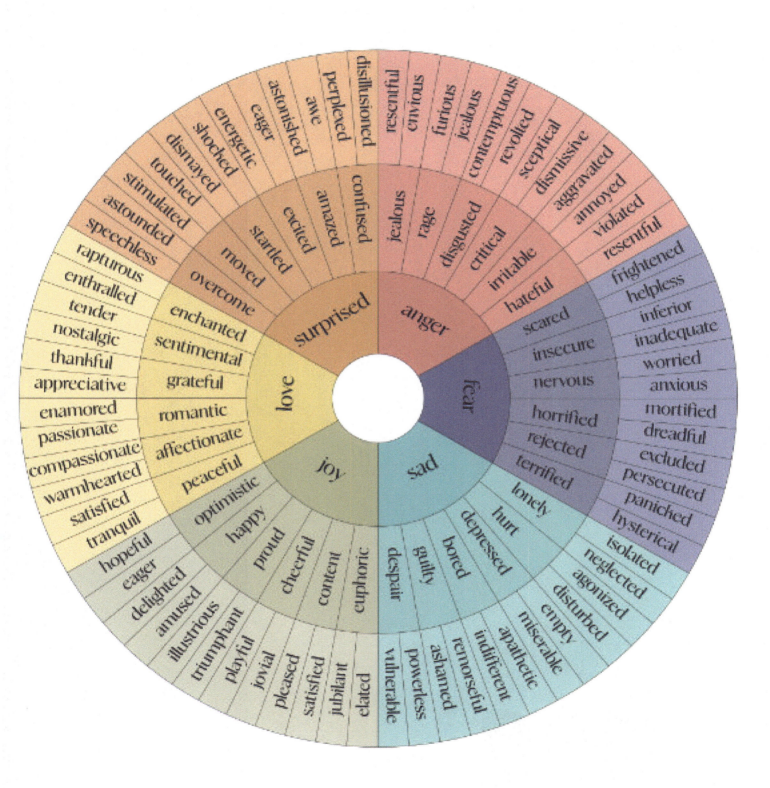

Spend some time studying the feelings wheel on the previous page. Which emotions have you experienced the most? Are there any you don't know? Look up some of the definitions. Expanding your emotion vocabulary can help you be more specific about how you're feeling. Write down or draw what you've learned. Can you create your own feelings wheel with emotions you experience frequently?

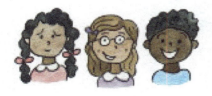

Draw a line between the two words that describe the same emotion.

sad   joyful

mad   gloomy

anxious   angry

happy   content

peaceful   worried

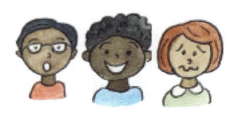

Draw a line between the matching face and emotion.

sad

happy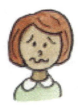

anxious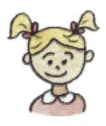

joyful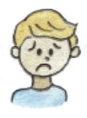

mad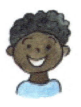

Write down the emotion that describes each person.

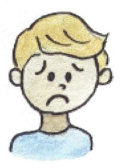 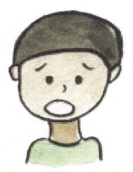

_____ _____

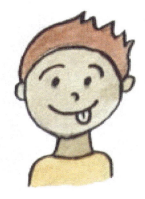 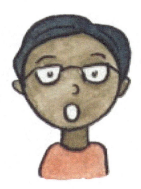

_____ _____

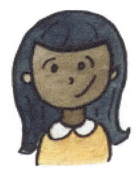 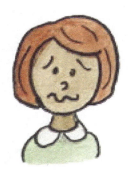

_____ _____

Write down the emotion that describes each person.

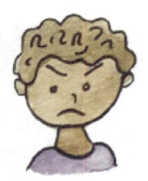 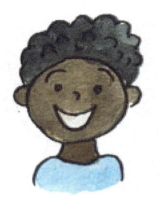

_____ _____

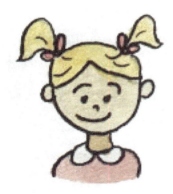 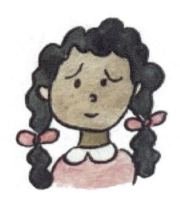

_____ _____

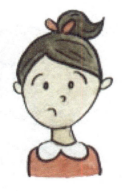 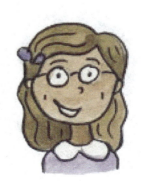

_____ _____

Our emotions often present themselves on a continuum, which means they range in their intensity. Match each emotion to either sad, happy, mad, or anxious.

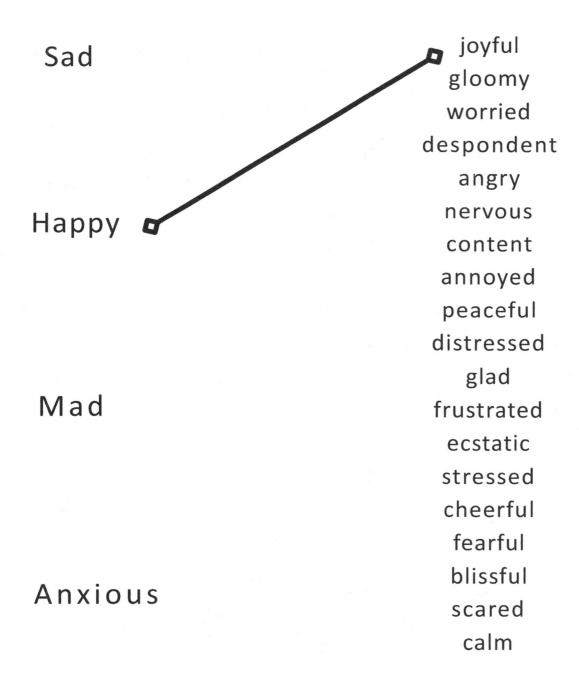

Emotions Word Find

```
G B D G J S R V H J U G D J H
M K L L D S Q C X C X H M O V
N G H A P P Y D S Y X D W Y V
Z A B D M K P U R I Y F S F J
W J K F Y B D G U L D Z X U Q
C F J S R U N W H M L P P L G
H H K Y U A H E Q A K K I O T
K H W G V D X C E S S A D E U
Q R O U T E F H M V C S A L P
R C R C R H H L E W Q O L D F
G G R E R A S X K L N B O C V
F G Y A E S B J L I U T V P G
Y H D S B U K L S C A R E D D
E L O N E L Y R K S F W D W M
D L E I I Y Y S D J K L P P B
```

Glad

Happy

Angry

Joyful

Sad

Scared

Loved

Lonely

Worry

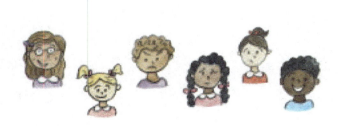

Name:_____

Feelings
Complete the crossword puzzle below

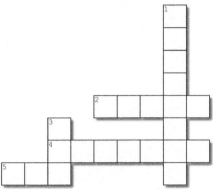

Created using the Crossword Maker on TheTeachersCorner.net

Across
2. when someone cares about us a great deal
4. when we feel worried about something
5. another word for angry

Down
1. when we appreciate what we have
3. another word for gloomy

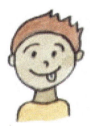
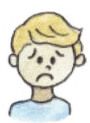
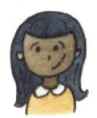
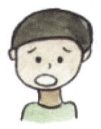
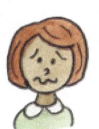
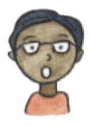

Why is it so important to learn how to manage our emotions? Look at this picture of the human body. Did you know many areas of our body are affected when we become upset? For example, we may have an upset stomach or clammy hands when we're anxious. Which parts of our body are affected when we're angry? How about sad? (Older students can spend some time researching some of the negative effects stress can have on our body). There is a vast amount of research that has been done on this subject. Take some time to explore some of the research about how our mental health and physical health are connected. There are helpful links in the appendix!

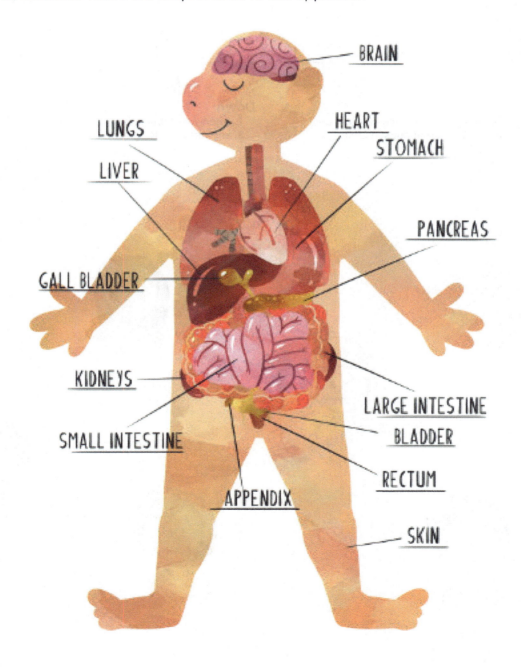

If your feelings were like the weather, what would they look like? Point to the picture that best describes how you feel today and discuss with your loved one. You can also draw what your mood would look like if it was weather! Would it look different than these pictures?

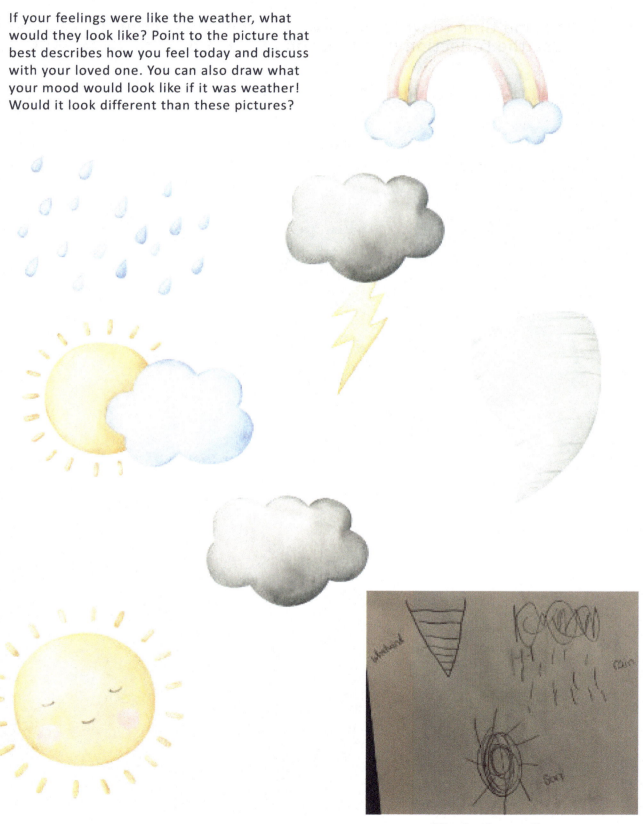

Elizabeth-age 7

Take some time to write or draw your thoughts about this chapter.
Use the reflection questions on the next page to guide you!

Reflection

What did you learn about emotions? How did this lesson add to the knowledge you already had about emotions? What questions do you still have? Name one thing you can do to begin identifying your emotions and expressing them in a healthy manner. Pick one emotion and look up the definition. Then find out what the Bible says about that particular emotion. What are the similarities and differences?

Chapter 2
Anger

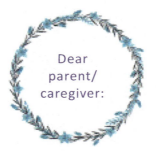

Dear parent/caregiver:

We've probably all experienced our child throwing themselves on the floor in a fit of anger. They are experiencing thoughts and emotions that are new to them and they are unable to express them in a healthy way. Unfortunately, not everyone was taught how to manage their emotions and they continue to struggle into adulthood. We can assist our own children in learning how to identify these feelings and cope with them in a healthy manner.

Anger is often a "secondary emotion" and may be experienced alongside other emotions, including but not limited to: anxiety, depression, grief, shame, embarrassment, feelings of failure or inadequacy, etc.

Anger may also be experienced when basic needs aren't being met, such as sleep, hunger, or thirst. When we think about anger as a signal that something is wrong, and not that our child is trying to be difficult, we find it easier to try to help them understand the root of their anger and what can be done. Children don't have the same vocabulary as adults and often have difficulty expressing themselves. They often express big emotions through their behavior. They might also express them through play.

The following exercises are designed for you to read and complete alongside your child. Let your child lead in how much you cover at once. Give them time to process each section before moving forward. You can pick and choose which section to begin first, but please read the corresponding parent/caregiver section before you begin working with your child on that particular issue.

If you feel that your child's anger is excessive, finding a play therapist in your area is highly encouraged. It is crucial that you, the parent/caregiver, are finding time for self-care as well.

Parent/caregiver journal exercise: What were you taught about anger? How did your parents express anger? What would you like to do differently? How did you express anger as a child? How about now? What do you need to work on?

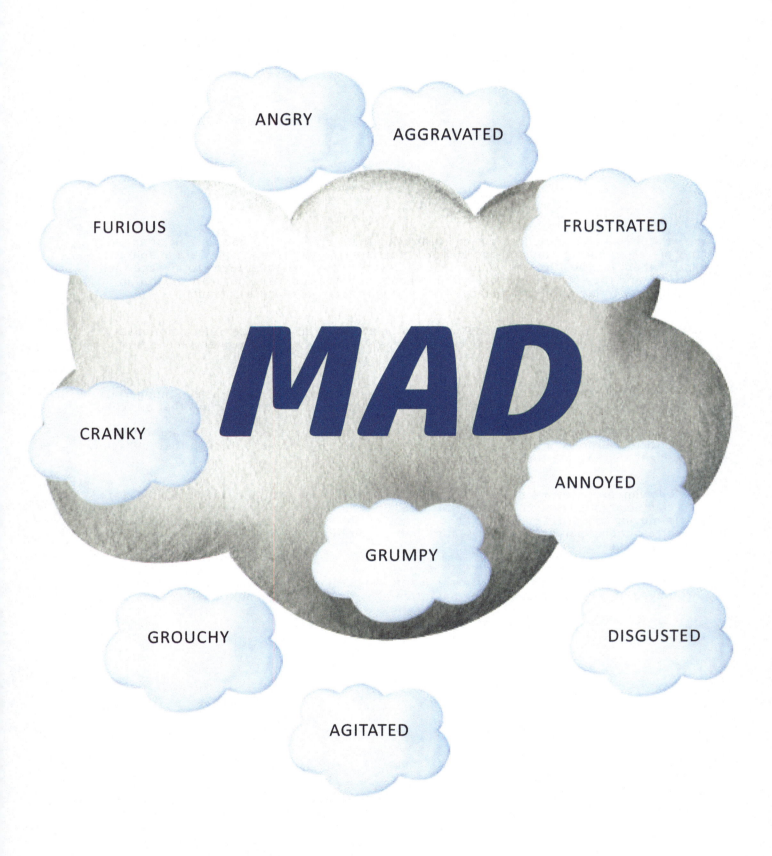

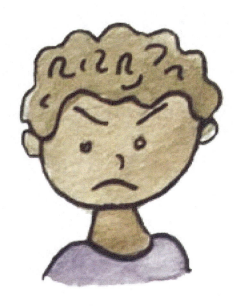

How do I know when I'm getting angry? I feel so mad. VERY VERY MAD!

My heart beats fast and my face feels hot and turns red.

I clench my jaw, I make a fist, I want to scream and shout!

My thoughts aren't kind and I want to say things I don't mean! Life just isn't fair!

I want to calm down, but I don't know how. I want to kick and bite and hit!

I want to stomp my feet and throw myself on the floor!

I just want to be alone. I have a frown on my face. I do not like feeling this way!

How can I calm down? What can I do? What does the Bible say?

"Anger will not help you live a good life as God wants." James 1:20 (ICB)

"My dear brothers, always be willing to listen and slow to speak. Do not become angry easily." James 1:19 (ICB)

When we feel these big emotions, we should remind ourselves we are normal. God made us to be able to feel and express so many emotions! This is one thing that makes us different from animals. We are created in God's image. During His time on Earth, Jesus experienced all of these emotions. He wants us to learn how to manage them. Anger doesn't help a situation, it makes it worse. It is important to remember that I am the only person in control of my behavior. The Bible is the best place we can learn about how God made us and how He wants us to live! Isn't it wonderful that He gave us something to help us grow?

Matthew 21 tells us about a time when Jesus became angry because the house of God was being disrespected. Read this passage and discuss what righteous anger means to you.

Draw Your Anger

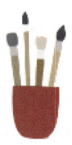

God has given us the ability to think creatively and use art to express ourselves. What does your anger look like? Does it have a certain shape? Color? What name would you give your anger?

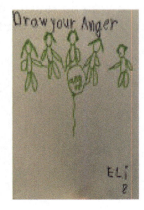

Eli-age 8

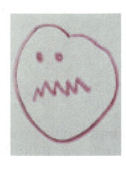

Elizabeth-age 7

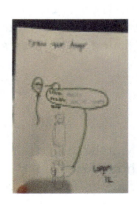

Logan-age 12

JOURNAL

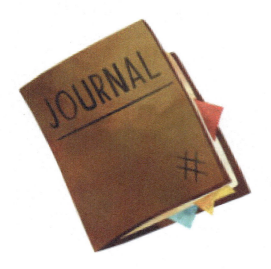

God gave us the gift of language as another way to express ourselves. Think about the last time you felt angry. What thoughts did you have? How did your body feel? What was happening in your environment?

_____

_____

_____

_____

Color where you feel anger in your body.

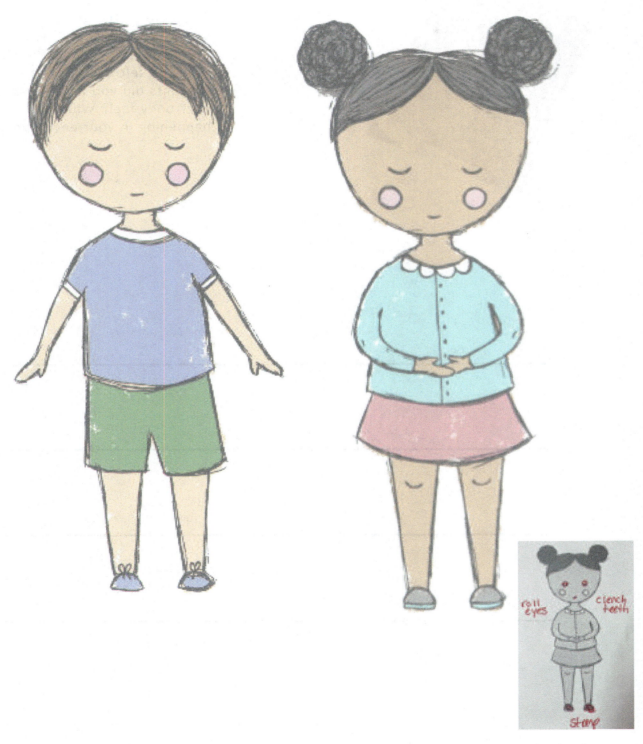

Elizabeth-7

How do we know that a thunderstorm is approaching our area? The sky gets dark, it gets windy, and the air changes. If we listen closely, we can hear thunder in the distance. We may even notice birds flying in a particular direction or notice our pets becoming upset.

We can also think about these early warning signs in reference to our anger. What are some early signs that you are getting angry?

Examples include: clenched fists, clenched jaw, hard breathing, pacing, fast heartbeat, fast thoughts, mean words, red face, shaking, grinding teeth, screaming, difficulty focusing, or hitting something. We may also withdraw and refuse to speak to anyone.

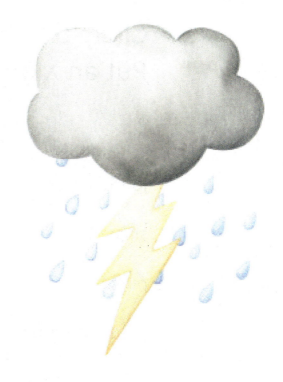

If we know our early warning signs, we can begin to manage our anger more effectively. (This analogy can also apply to our anxiety or worry).

Write down your early warning signs of anger here:

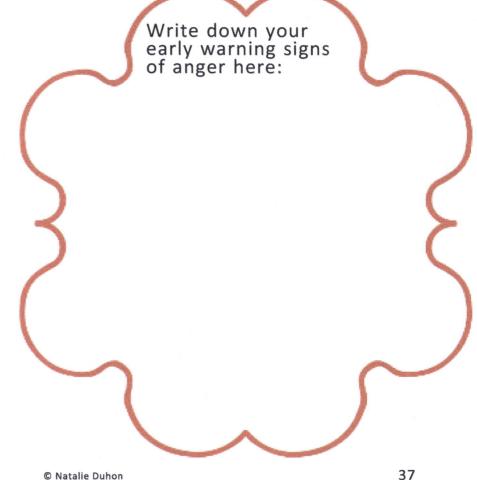

Circle the behaviors that are okay. Put an X on the ones that are not.

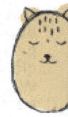

- hit
- journal
- slap
- punch
- break something
- talk to someone
- yell
- pray
- listen to soothing music
- throw things
- denial (pretend my anger isn't there)

- take a bath
- go to a quiet room
- count to 10
- ask an adult for help
- hit
- hug a stuffed animal
- bite
- scream and shout
- take a deep breath
- cry

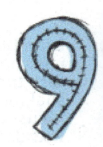

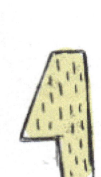
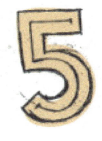
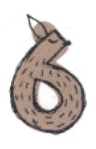
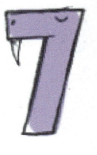

© Natalie Duhon

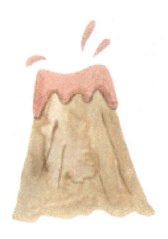

It's okay to feel angry. If we try to hide it or stuff our anger, we will make it worse. Then we will explode like a volcano. Have you ever felt that way? Our feelings are okay. Certain behaviors are NOT okay. God gave us many emotions and it's okay to feel them. How we act is different. It is NOT okay to hurt myself or someone else. It is NOT okay to destroy things.

Remember-crying IS okay!!!

It can be helpful to look at our anger on a continuum. What are some things that trigger our anger? (Example: someone takes a toy from us)

10-worst anger ever

9

8

7

6-pretty angry

5

4-getting annoyed

3

2

1

0-calm, no anger

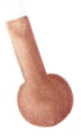

If your anger had a temperature, how high would it be? How can you cool down?

What are your anger triggers (thoughts or situations that cause you to become angry)? Write or draw them here. Then rate them using the scale on the next page.

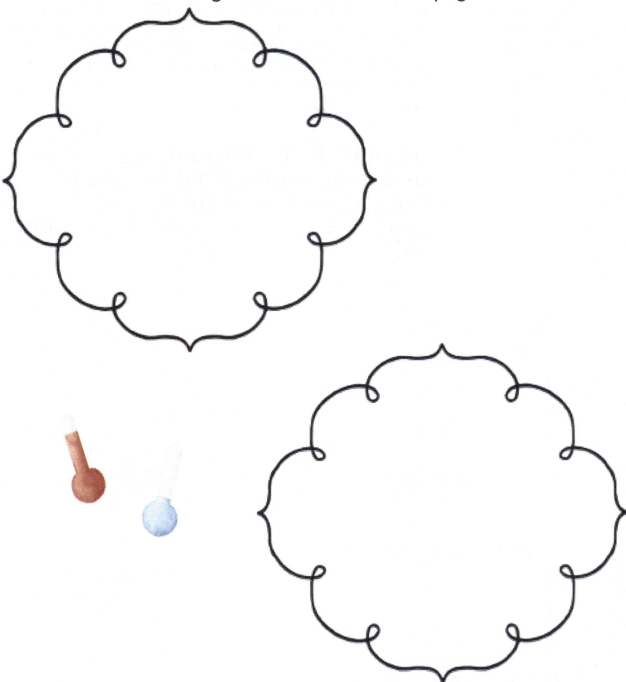

10-worst anger ever

9

8

7

6

5

4

3

2

1

0-calm, no anger

On this thermometer, write down some ways you can "cool down" when you're angry.

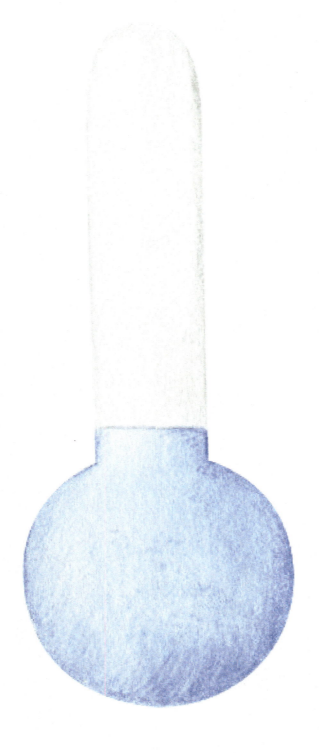

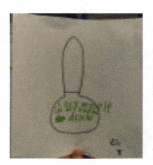

Eli-age 8

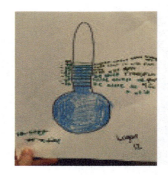

Logan-age 12

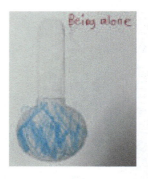

Elizabeth-age 7

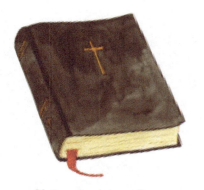

In the Bible, we are instructed to hide the Word of God in our hearts. We can do this by memorizing Scripture. When we do this, it will be easier to remember when we have BIG feelings. (Singing can also help us memorize Scripture). Copy the following verse and then discuss what it means to you.

"A gentle answer will calm a person's anger. But an unkind answer will cause more anger." Proverbs 15:1 (ICB)

_____

_____

_____

_____

_____

_____

Thank you God, for the air in my lungs. Thank you for the ability to think and feel, which are the things you do too. Please help me remember to be quick to listen and slow to become angry. Please help me see how my anger hurts others, myself, and you. Amen

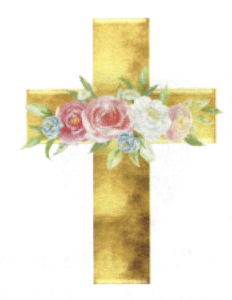

Add your prayer here:

_____

_____

_____

_____

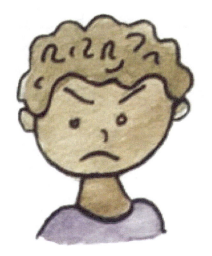

Think about the last time you were angry. What happened? What was your role in the situation? What could you have done differently? What did you do that helped the situation? What can you do in the future? Remember, the only person who can control your anger is YOU! However, you can always ask God for help!

_____

_____

_____

_____

"A foolish person loses his temper. But a wise person controls his anger." Proverbs 29:11

Take some time to write or draw your thoughts about this chapter.
Use the reflection questions on the next page to guide you!

Reflection

What did you learn about anger? How did this lesson add to the knowledge you already had about anger? What questions do you still have? Name one thing you can do to begin identifying your anger and expressing it in a healthy manner. Look up the definition of anger, then find out what the Bible says. What are the similarities and differences?

Chapter 3
Anxiety

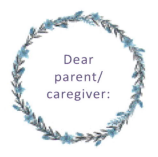

Dear parent/caregiver:

Most, if not all of us have experienced anxiety at some point. It's helpful if we look at anxiety on a continuum, from mildly concerned all the way to full-blown panic. I will list some commonly experienced anxiety symptoms here, but please be aware that this is not an exhaustive list.

Symptoms may include: frequent worry, upset stomach, muscle tension/aches, avoidance of stressful situations, poor focus, headache, nervousness, fast heartbeat, appetite or sleep disturbance, restlessness or shakiness, and irritability. In children, a change in behavior can be an early sign of anxiety. This can include crying spells, tantrums, increased anxiety in social situations, and fear of embarrassment.

These physical sensations can cause our children great distress if they don't understand them. Chronic stress can be detrimental to our health, so it is important that we learn healthy ways to manage it. We can teach our children to notice what is happening in their bodies when they are upset. It takes time and practice, but even young children can learn this important skill.

There are many helpful videos and apps that teach deep breathing, guided imagery, and "progressive muscle relaxation." These skills can be helpful in managing feelings of worry and anxiety. Preview them before watching with your child to ensure they align with your values and beliefs. These techniques have been researched extensively, with fantastic results.

https://www.therapistaid.com/ is a great place to find out more information.

Only a qualified mental health professional or medical doctor can make an accurate diagnosis. If you are concerned about the severity of your child's anxiety (or your own), please obtain professional help.

Journal for parents/caregivers: What has been your experience with anxiety? What are your early warning signs of anxiety? How have you managed anxiety in the past (helpful and unhelpful)? How do you manage anxiety now?

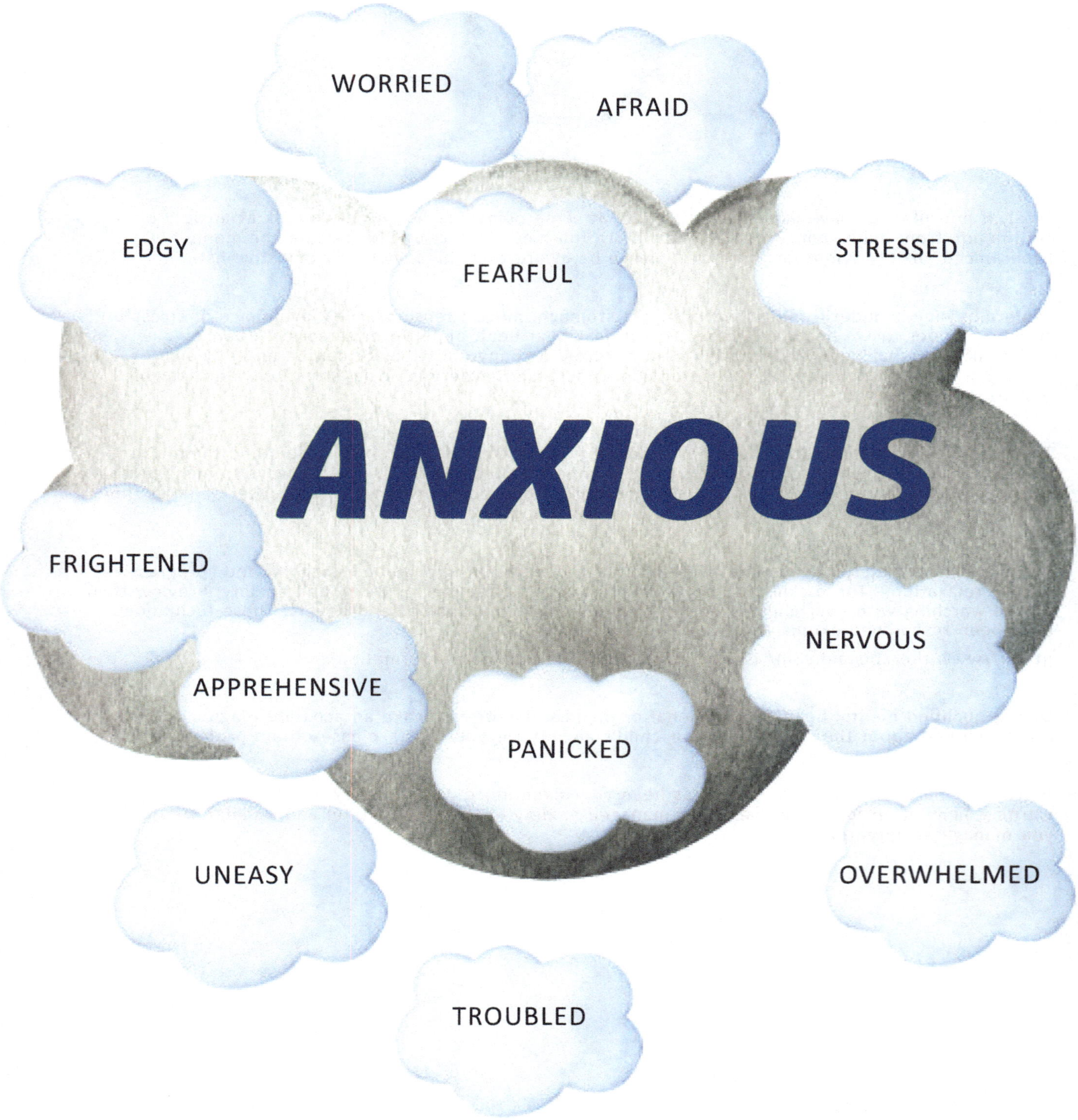

ANXIOUS

- WORRIED
- AFRAID
- EDGY
- FEARFUL
- STRESSED
- FRIGHTENED
- APPREHENSIVE
- NERVOUS
- PANICKED
- UNEASY
- OVERWHELMED
- TROUBLED

Sometimes I feel shy and can't talk. Sometimes I want to run and hide. My thoughts go super fast and I have trouble focusing. I feel confused and can't think straight. Sometimes I get so restless, I need to run as fast as I can. I can't sit still, even though I try. I'm full of energy and I need to let it out. Why is my heart beating so fast? Why am I sweating so much? My knees are knocking together and my voice feels shaky. Other times, I need to do something that helps me feel calm, but what can I do?

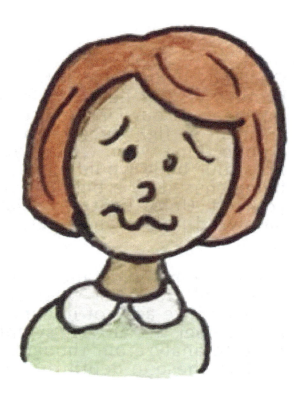

I think of all sorts of things. I worry that I won't have fun at the birthday party. I worry that I'll have a bad dream. I worry that my friend won't like me anymore. What can I do with all of these feelings?

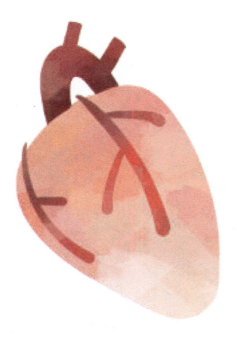

Our bodies are made with an internal stress response that is designed to protect us from danger. Unfortunately, we sometimes think or feel that we are in danger when we are not, and our body responds accordingly. (Parent/caregiver, you may want to help your older children research this further). It's amazing how God created our bodies!

Our body is designed with a "fight or flight" response that serves to protect us. Our heart begins beating faster and blood rushes from our head to our large muscles, enabling us to temporarily be stronger to fight or able to run faster than we normally can. This is a good thing when we are actually in danger! If your house was on fire, your body would allow you to get to safety quickly. If you were being chased by a big dog, your body would allow you to protect yourself. Unfortunately anxiety might also cause us to become paralyzed in fear and "freeze."

There are many instances where our "fight or flight" response is beneficial. However, when we experience those reactions in our body and we are not in danger, it can pose some problems. (Remember the anxiety symptoms we discussed)? That's when we need to analyze our thoughts and use our coping skills. (We will explore these in depth throughout this book!)

Prayer: Thank you, God, for creating my mind and body with the ability to protect myself and others. Please help me discern true danger versus worry and anxiety.

Remember the thunderstorm analogy we used when thinking about our early warning signs of anger? Let's do the same for anxiety. What are some early warning signs that you are becoming worried or anxious? Write them here!

Ways to cope with anxiety

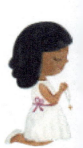

Talk to someone	Play a game
Deep breathing	Grounding exercises
Listen to music	Read my Bible
Pray	Journal
Pet an animal	Praise God for His creation
Draw or color	Use progressive muscle relaxation
Sing	Word/number puzzles
Dance	Exercise
Go outside	Read

Pretend to blow bubbles/candles

Sensory items: clay, sand, finger paint, rice, etc.

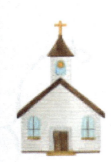

Add your own:

_____

_____

Draw Your Worry

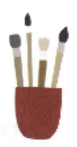

God has given us the ability to think creatively and use art to express ourselves. What does your worry look like? Does it have a certain shape? Color? What name would you give your worry?

Color where you feel worry in your body.

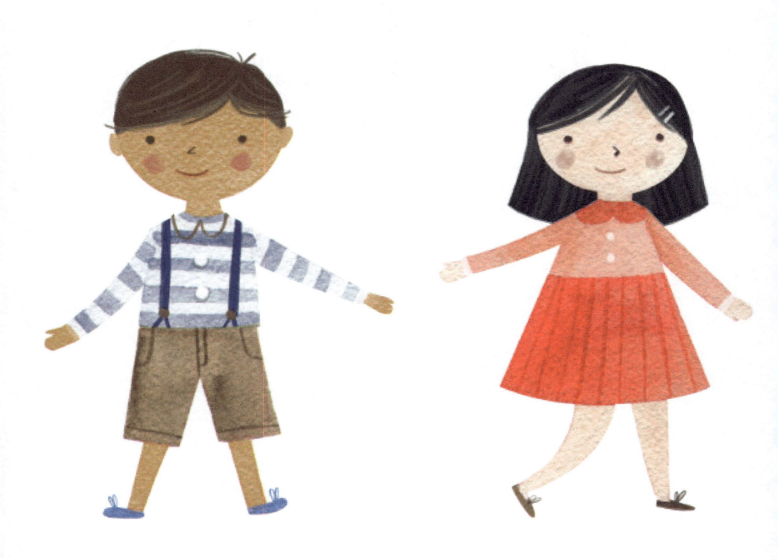

What does the Bible say about worry?

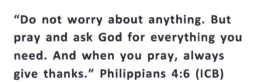

"When five sparrows are sold, they cost only two pennies. But God does not forget any of them. Yes, God even knows how many hairs you have on your head. Don't be afraid. You are worth much more than many sparrows." Luke 12:6-8 (ICB)

"Do not worry about anything. But pray and ask God for everything you need. And when you pray, always give thanks." Philippians 4:6 (ICB)

"Jesus said, "Don't let your hearts be troubled. Trust in God. And trust in me." John 14:1 (ICB)

"God did not give us a spirit that makes us afraid. He gave us a spirit of power and love and self-control." 2 Timothy 1:7 (ICB)

"So don't worry, because I am with you. Don't be afraid, because I am your God. I will make you strong and will help you. I will support you with my right hand that saves you." Isaiah 41:10 (ICB)

© Natalie Duhon

What can I do about my anxiety?

There are specific steps I can take to begin combating my anxiety.

1. Be as specific as possible about the current problem. What thoughts do I have about it? Are they helping me or causing me anguish (emotional suffering)? *We will learn more about our thoughts a bit later.

2. What are some steps I can take to resolve the problem? How can I take action right now? Who can I ask for help? What resources do I need? Who are some safe people I can talk to? How have I coped so far? Have my actions helped the situation or made it worse?

3. Have I encountered a similar problem in the past? How did I cope then? Was there anything that helped that will also help me now?

4. What are some things about my problem that are out of my control? This is the hard part! Let's pray and ask God for help letting go of the things that are out of our control.

5. After praying, use some relaxation techniques. (We'll cover those soon! Feel free to skip ahead to the relaxation chapter). Remember, it takes practice!

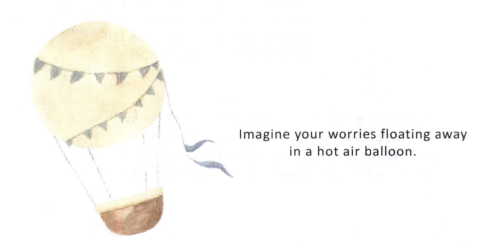

Imagine your worries floating away in a hot air balloon.

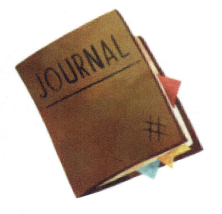

Read the book of Jonah together. God clearly spoke to Jonah about what He wanted Jonah to do, but Jonah ran away. He was experiencing fear instead of relying on God. How can you relate to this story? What happened when Jonah trusted God? What happened when he didn't? What happens when we trust God? What happens when we don't? Journal your thoughts here.

___

___

___

___

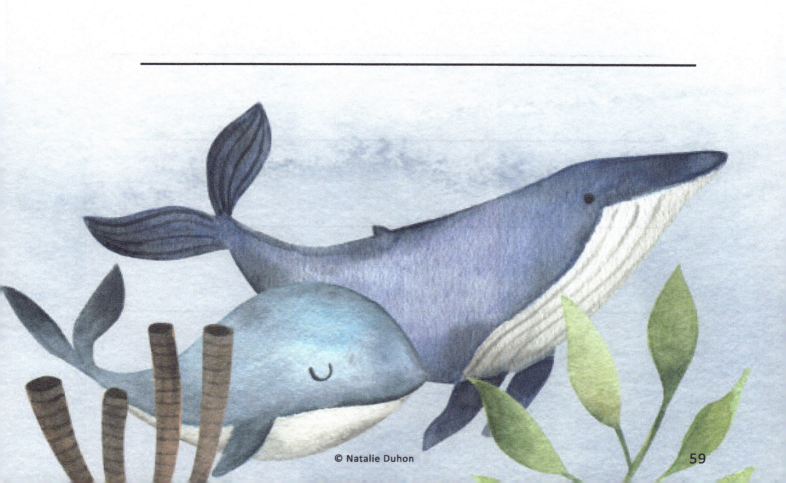

Hymns for Worry

It is Well with My Soul (Research the history of this hymn. Share with older children if appropriate).
I Sing the Mighty Power of God
Amazing Grace
Be Not Afraid
Blessed Assurance
How Great Thou Art

Write down the lyrics of your favorite hymn. How can it provide you comfort during difficult times?

_____

_____

_____

_____

JOURNAL

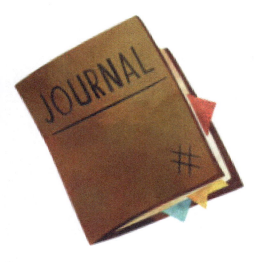

God gave us the gift of language as another way to express ourselves. Think about the last time you felt worry. What thoughts did you have? How did your body feel? What was happening in your environment? Were you worried about something in your control or out of your control?

_____

_____

_____

_____

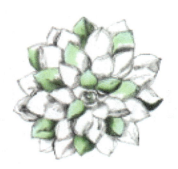

What are some things that might cause you to feel worry?

- riding a bike for the first time
- swimming lessons
- the dark
- meeting someone new
- heights
- bad weather
- animals
- doctor/dentist
- being alone
- large crowds
- change

Do any of these cause you to feel worried or anxious? What would you add to the list? Write them down here.

Take some time to write or draw your thoughts about this chapter.
Use the reflection questions on the next page to guide you!

Reflection

What did you learn about anxiety/worry?

How did this lesson add to the knowledge you already had about anxiety/worry?

What questions do you still have?

Name one thing you can do to begin identifying your anxiety/worry and expressing it in a healthy manner.

Look up the definition of anxiety/worry, then find out what the Bible says. What are the similarities and differences?

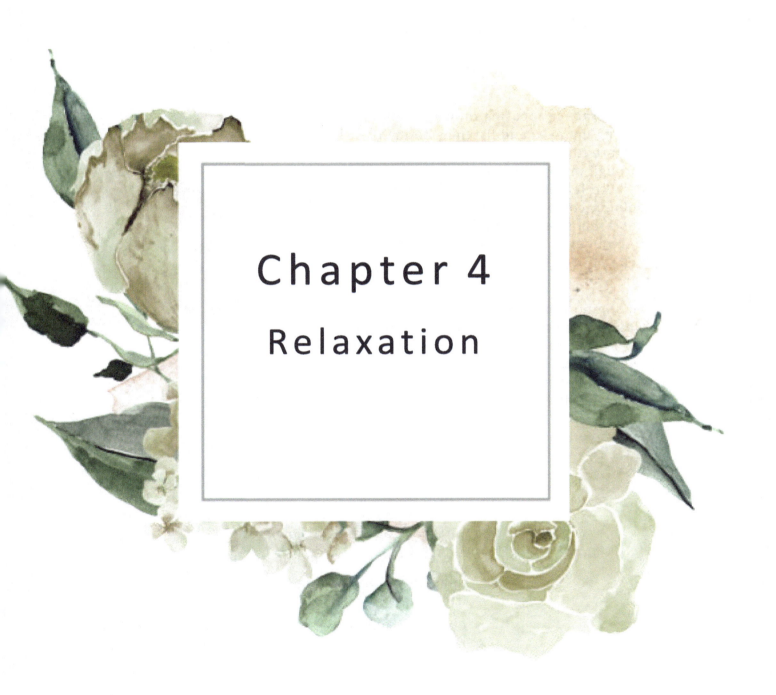

Chapter 4
Relaxation

Deep Breathing

When we worry a lot, we tend to take shorter and more shallow breaths. This makes it hard for us to take in enough oxygen. We need oxygen to live because of the unique way God designed us!

I can practice focusing on my breathing by closing my eyes and listening to my breath. I can breathe in through my nose and out through my mouth. I can put my hand on my belly to feel it move. This helps me know I'm doing it correctly! If I do this a few times, my heart will stop beating so fast and I will start to feel better. This may take some practice, but I can do it!

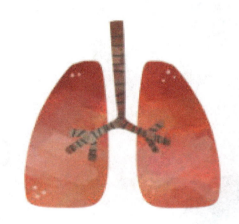

*It's important to practice deep breathing when you're calm. This will help your body learn what to do when you become anxious or angry. Be careful not to take too many deep breaths at once. This may cause you to hyperventilate! (Hyperventilation is when you breathe too fast and get too much oxygen. This makes you feel dizzy).

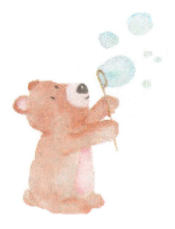

Ways to practice deep breathing:

Pretend you're blowing out the candles on your birthday cake, but in slow motion!

Pretend you're blowing up a balloon!

Imagine you're blowing bubbles or go outside and do it!

Count the number of breaths you take. You will notice that focusing on your breath helps you relax.

What happens to your body when you focus on your breath? (Your shoulders and neck might loosen, your breathing should slow down).

© Natalie Duhon

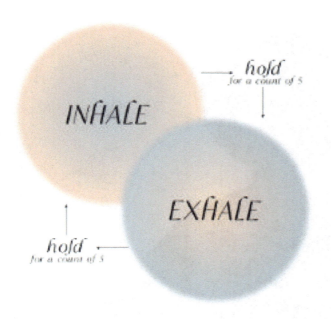

These posters can be laminated and used as a reminder of ways to cope with anxiety.

Tips to calm *yourself* down

- Practice deep breathing
- Challenge your thoughts
- Visualize yourself calm
- Listen to music
- Take a bath
- Light a candle
- Write it down
- Change your focus

What did you notice about deep breathing? Circle the parts of your body that relaxed.

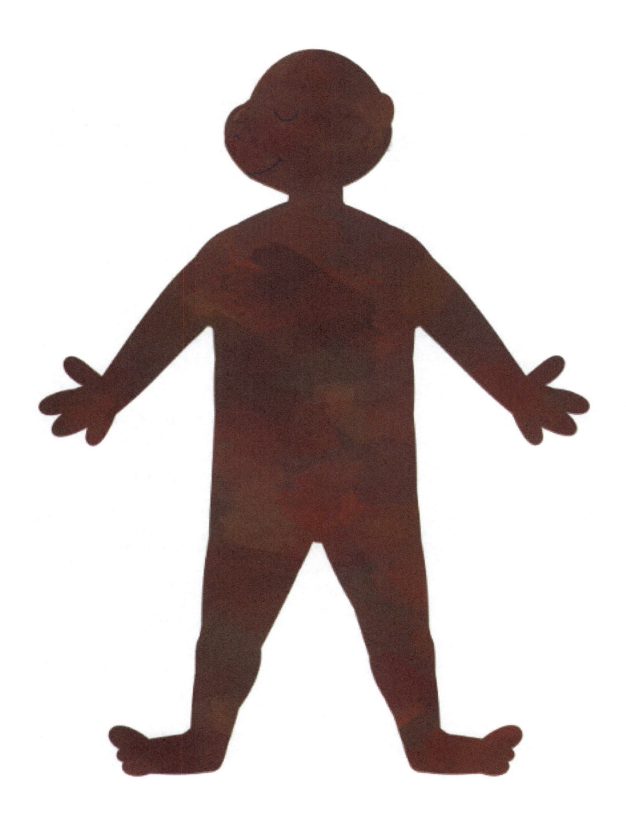

Grounding

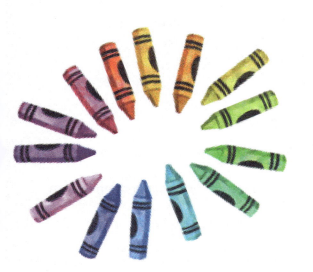

Grounding is a fancy term for using your five senses to focus on what's going on in your life right now. Do you remember your five senses? God made them for us to experience His world! They are sight, sound, taste, touch, and smell. How do they help us? You can use your five senses to help you focus on what's right in front of you instead of worries that are out of your control.

What do I see? What are the colors, shapes, lines, patterns, or curves?

What do I hear? Loud or soft sounds? Nature? Music? Traffic? Dogs barking?

What do I smell? Pleasant or unpleasant?

What do I taste? Pleasant or unpleasant? Sweet, salty, bitter, sour?

What do I feel on my skin? Wind? Hot or cold? Soft or hard? Smooth or rough? Warmth from the sunshine?

One benefit of grounding is that it can be used anywhere, at anytime. It is a great skill to help us focus on the present. This will allow us to stay calm so we can figure out a good way to solve our problem.

I can use my five senses to feel better when I'm worried! They can also help with other feelings, such as sadness or anger! Circle the ones that are most helpful to you. Feel free to add your own!

warm bath with bubbles that smell good	pet an animal
warm, soft blanket or stuffed animal	hug a loved one
pretty picture or painting	close your eyes and take a deep breath
clay	talk to someone you love
music	spend time in God's creation
nature sounds	sing
warm sunshine or cool breeze	play an instrument
pleasant smells	create something
hot chocolate	fingerpaint
garden	pick/smell flowers

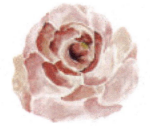
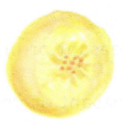
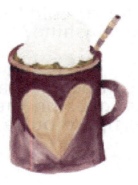
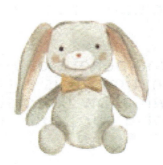

Let's practice using your five senses! Sit down quietly for a few minutes and focus on one sense at a time. Then write down or draw your experience.

SIGHT (see)

TOUCH (feel)

SOUND (hear)

SMELL

TASTE

Take away one of your five senses and try to imagine life without it. Draw, journal, or tell a loved one about your experience.

SIGHT
(blindfold)

TOUCH
(use gloves)

SOUND
(use earplugs)

SMELL
(plug your nose)

TASTE
(bland food)

Thank you, God, for my five senses. Please help me be more aware of these beautiful gifts you have given me to experience life more fully.

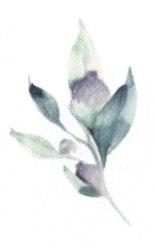

Use your five senses to appreciate the beauty God has created for us. On a separate sheet of paper, draw/paint a picture of something in God's creation. Thank God for the beauty He gives us every day. Journal about or draw the night sky. Describe the beach, a mountain, a forest, or think about the most beautiful place in God's creation. Although we live in a broken world, we can see God's hand everywhere. Can you imagine what Heaven will look like?

"Using His wisdom, the Lord made the earth. Using his understanding, He set the sky in place. Using His knowledge, He made rivers flow from underground springs. And He made the clouds drop rain on the earth." Proverbs 3:19-20 (ICB)

"But as it is written in the Scriptures: "No one has ever seen this. No one has ever heard about it. No one has ever imagined what God has prepared for those who love Him." 1 Cor 2:9 (ICB)

Think about incorporating nature study in your home. How does studying God's creation help improve your mood?

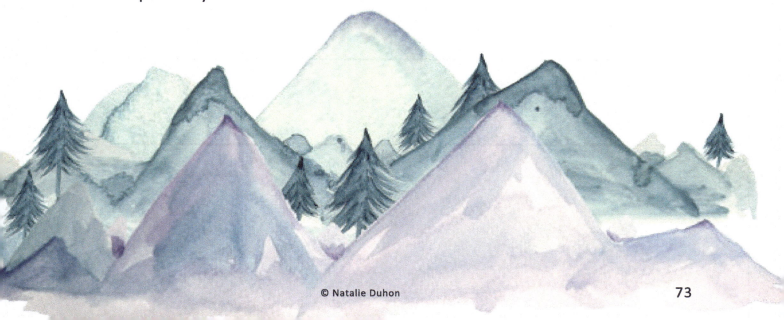

© Natalie Duhon

Copy and memorize the following Bible verse:

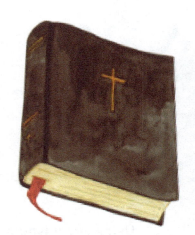

"Be still and know that I am God."
Psalm 46:10 (ICB)

_____

_____

_____

_____

Take some time to write or draw your thoughts about this chapter.
Use the reflection questions on the next page to guide you!

Reflection

What did you learn about relaxation? How did this lesson add to the knowledge you already had? What questions do you still have? How can you implement some of these relaxation activities into your life? How can they be beneficial? What does the Bible say about rest?

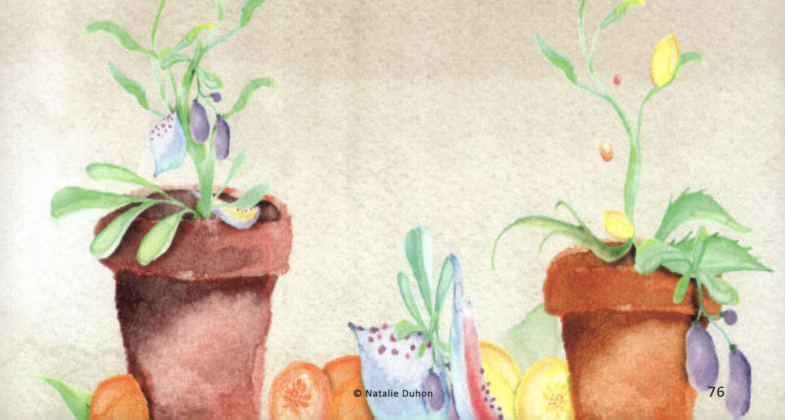

Chapter 5
Sadness

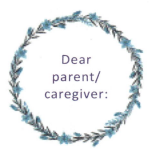

Dear parent/caregiver:

Sadness is a normal part of being human. God created us with the ability to experience numerous emotions, and it's important to know what the Bible says about them. Not all sadness will lead to depression, but it is helpful to be aware of some warning signs. Signs of depression include loss of interest, low energy, withdrawal from normal activities, increased crying spells, appetite disturbance, and difficulty functioning. (For more information about depression, consult the appendix for parent resources).

If your child is experiencing thoughts of hurting him/herself or someone else, contact a local professional immediately. Any comments related to self-harm or harming others should be taken seriously. This book is not intended to diagnose/treat severe mental health concerns and is not a replacement for therapy or medical treatment.

Mothers: it is important to be aware of your own mental health, especially while pregnant and after giving birth. Talk to your medical provider about signs of postpartum depression, anxiety, and psychosis. We are better mothers when we take care of ourselves too. Your OBGYN is a great resource. In some situations, medication and/or therapy may be necessary.

Journal for parents/caregiver: What has been your experience with depression? What are your early warning signs of sadness or depression? How have you managed depression in the past (helpful and unhelpful)? How do you manage depression and sadness now?

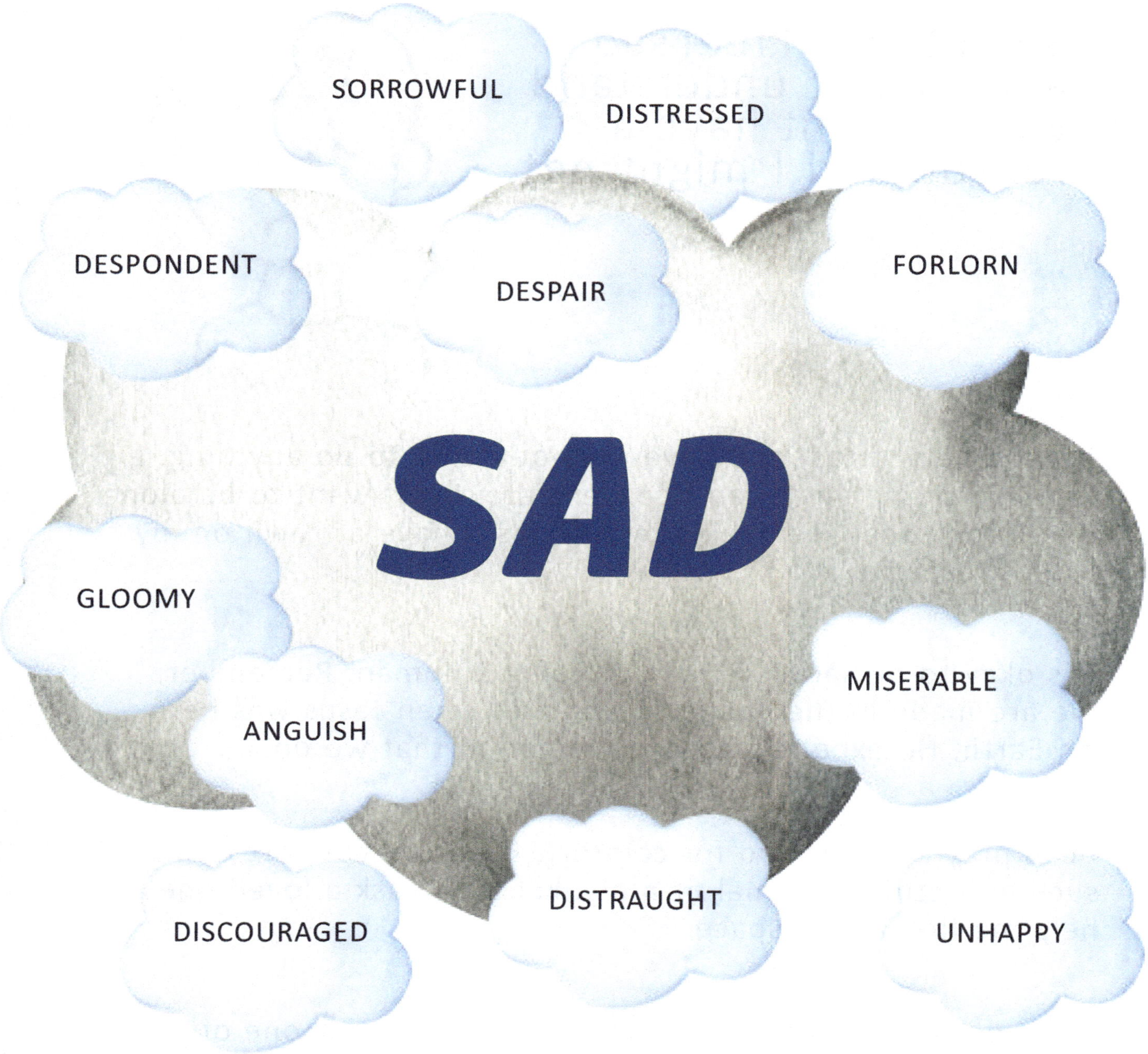

SAD

- SORROWFUL
- DISTRESSED
- DESPONDENT
- DESPAIR
- FORLORN
- GLOOMY
- ANGUISH
- MISERABLE
- DISCOURAGED
- DISTRAUGHT
- UNHAPPY

Sometimes I feel sad and I don't understand why. I might have a reason and I might not.

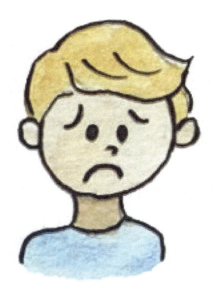

I feel empty, tired, and have no motivation to do anything. I feel like crying and I can't concentrate. I just want to be alone and I don't feel like seeing my friends. I have a frown on my face. What can I do?

It's okay to be sad, it is part of being a human. Remember, we are made in the image of God and when Jesus was here on Earth, He experienced every emotion that we do.

I can pray and ask God for comfort. I can use comfort items such as a stuffed animal or a blanket. I can ask a loved one to help me find a safe space.

What does the Bible teach us about sadness? Pick one of the following verses to write down and memorize. (Or choose your own!)

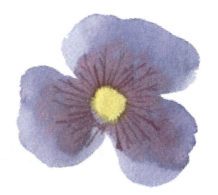

"Why am I so sad? Why am I so upset? I should put my hope in God. I should keep praising Him, my Savior and my God." Psalm 42:11 (ICB)

"Come near to God, and God will come near to you." James 4:8 (ICB)

"Crying may last for a night. But joy comes in the morning." Psalm 30:5 (ICB)

"The Lord is close to the brokenhearted. He saves those whose spirits have been crushed." Psalm 34:18 (ICB)

Revelation 21:3-4 (ICB) promises: **"Now God's home is with men. He will live with them, and they will be His people. God Himself will be with them and will be their God. He will wipe away every tear from their eyes. There will be no more death, sadness, crying, or pain. All the old ways are gone."**

John 14:1-4 (ICB) gives us comfort: **"Jesus said, "Don't let your hearts be troubled. Trust in God. And trust in Me. There are many rooms in my Father's house. I would not tell you this if it were not true. I am going there to prepare a place for you. After I go and prepare a place for you, I will come back. Then I will take you to be with me so that you may be where I am. You know the way to the place where I am going."**

© Natalie Duhon

Draw Your Sadness

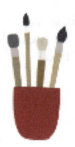 God has given us the ability to think creatively and use art to express ourselves. What does your sadness look like? Does it have a certain shape? Color? What name would you give your sadness?

JOURNAL

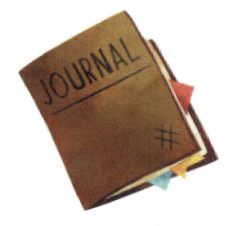

God gave us the gift of language as another way to express ourselves. Think about the last time you felt sad. What thoughts did you have? How did your body feel? What was happening in your environment?

_____

_____

_____

_____

"You changed my sorrow into dancing. You took away my rough cloth, which shows sadness, and clothed me in happiness." Psalm 30:11 (ICB)

Color where you feel sadness in your body.

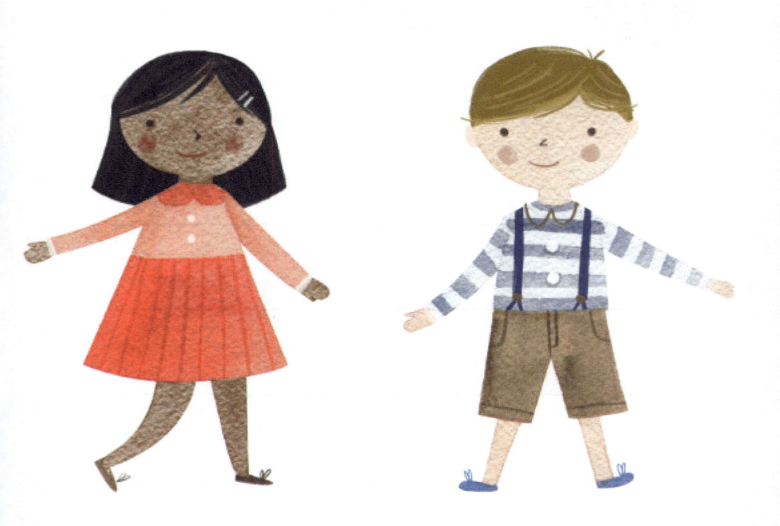

Take some time to write or draw your thoughts about this chapter.
Use the reflection questions on the next page to guide you!

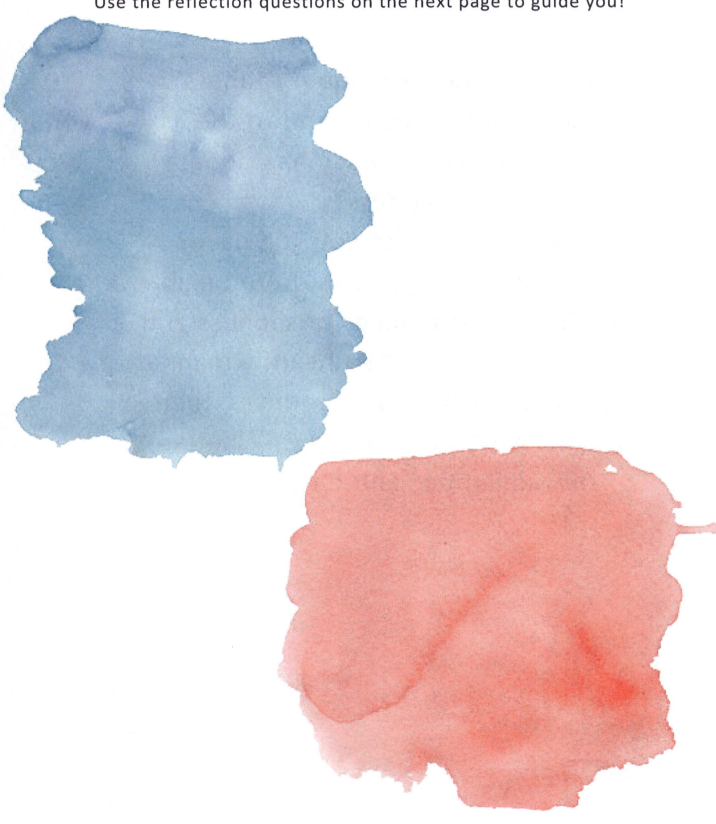

Reflection

What did you learn about sadness?
How did this lesson add to the knowledge you already had about sadness?
What questions do you still have?
Name one thing you can do to begin identifying your feelings of sadness and expressing sadness in a healthy manner.
Look up the definition of sadness, then find out what the Bible says. What are the similarities and differences?

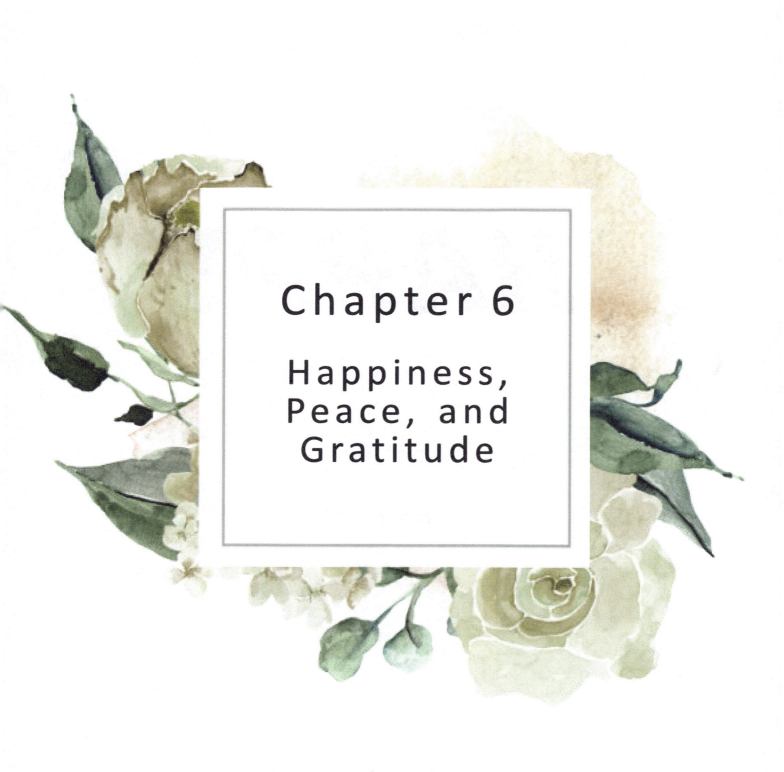

Chapter 6

Happiness, Peace, and Gratitude

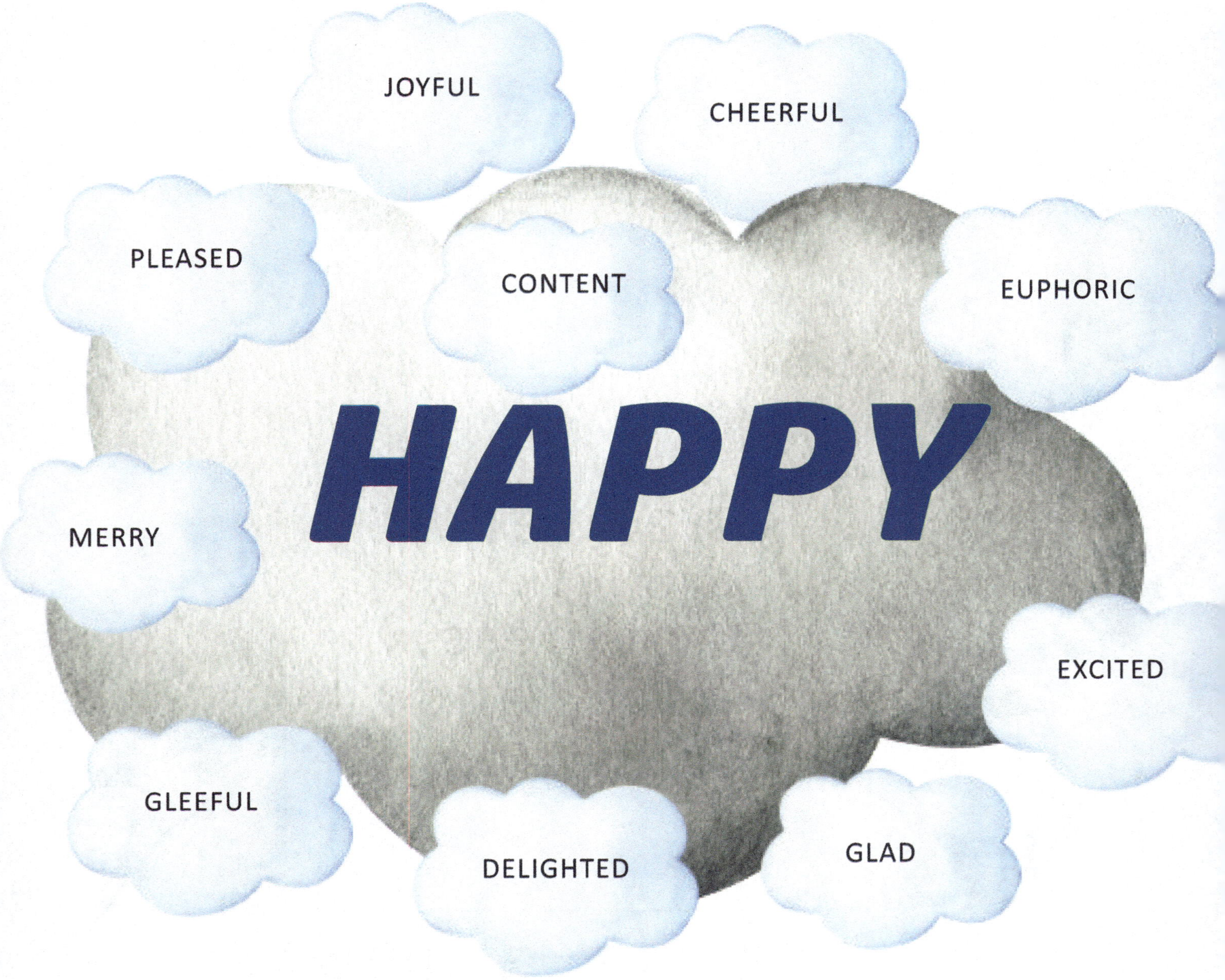

HAPPY

- JOYFUL
- CHEERFUL
- PLEASED
- CONTENT
- EUPHORIC
- MERRY
- EXCITED
- GLEEFUL
- DELIGHTED
- GLAD

When I'm happy, I feel like smiling and I don't have anything to be upset about! What does the Bible say about happiness?

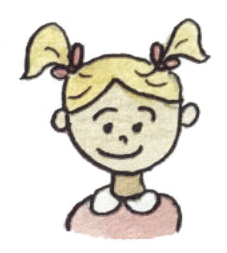

Draw a memory that makes you happy. Where can you see God working in your life then and now? Using clay, create something that makes you happy.

"I will go to the altar of God, to God who is my joy and happiness. I will praise you with a harp, God, my God." Psalm 43:4 (ICB)

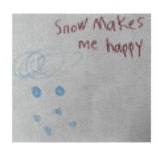

Elizabeth-age 7

"Happy is the person who finds wisdom. And happy is the person who gets understanding." Proverbs 3:13 (ICB)

Draw your favorite animal. The Bible says we should care for God's creatures. He expects us to be kind to them. Having a pet or visiting animals can help us feel happy and give us a sense of purpose. Animals are a fantastic way to improve our mental health. (Older children might want to research the benefits pets have on mental health).

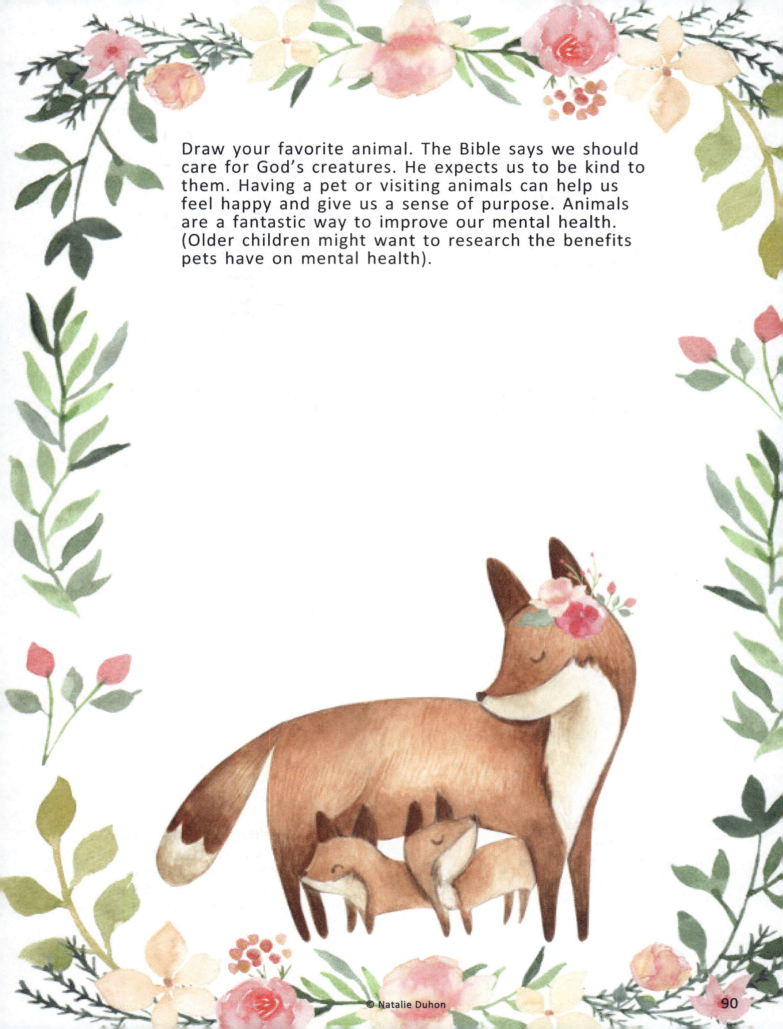

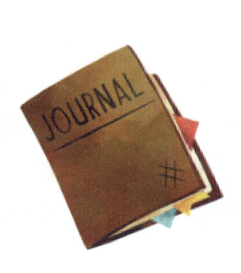
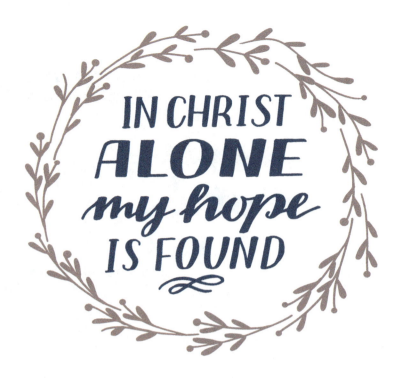

What does this verse mean to you? Journal your thoughts here or discuss with your loved one.

_____

_____

_____

_____

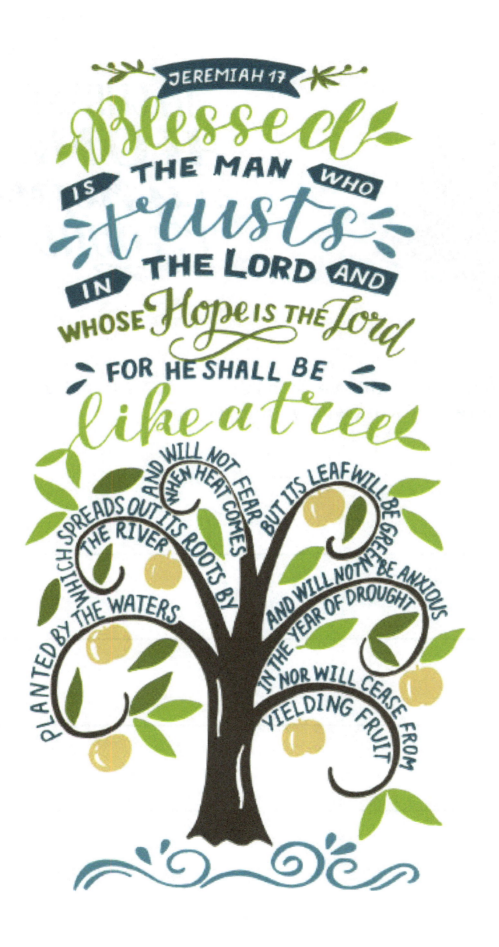

THANKFUL

VALUE

PRAISE

GRATITUDE

GRATEFUL

RECOGNIZE

THANKSGIVING

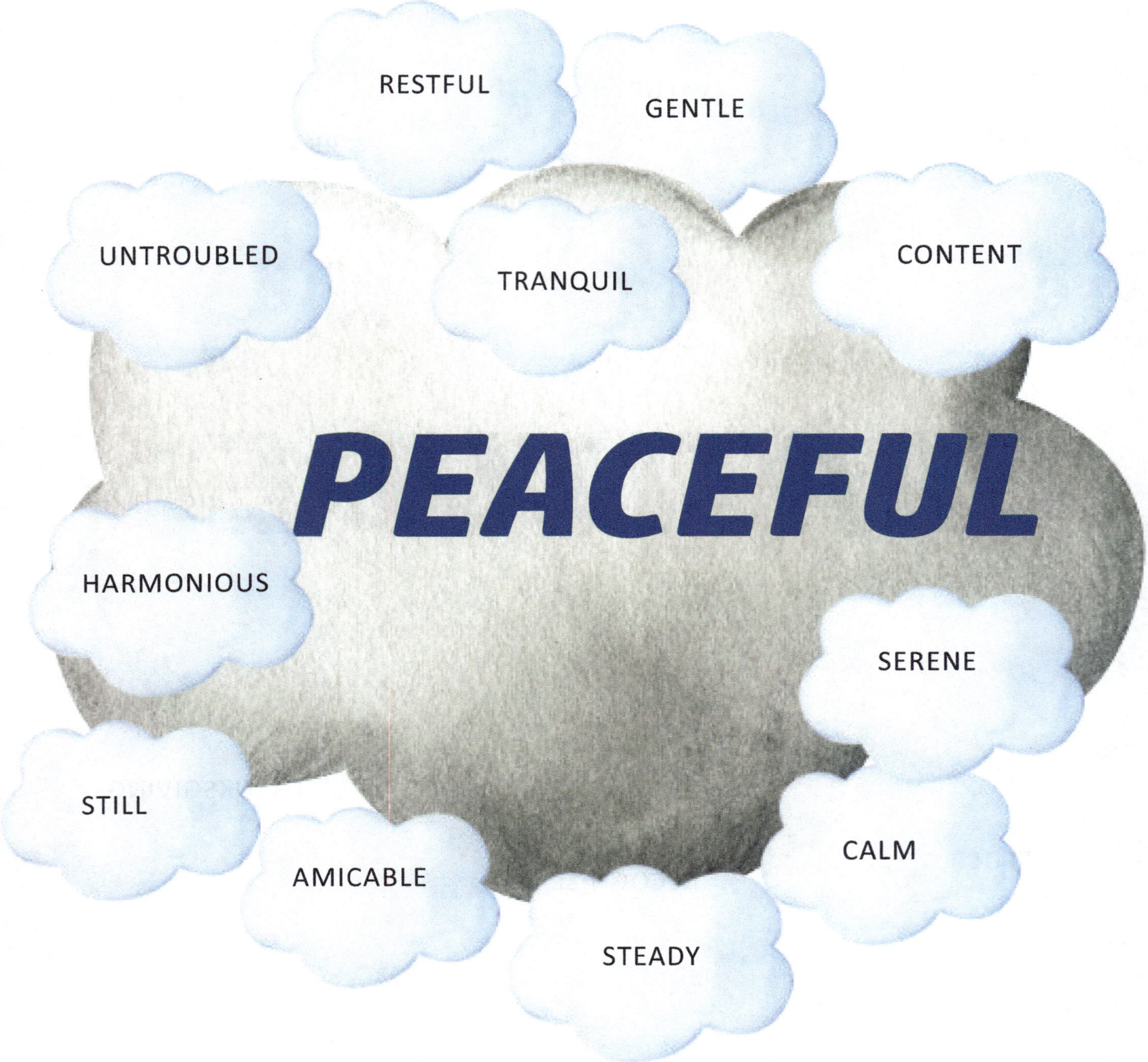

PEACEFUL

- RESTFUL
- GENTLE
- UNTROUBLED
- TRANQUIL
- CONTENT
- HARMONIOUS
- SERENE
- STILL
- CALM
- AMICABLE
- STEADY

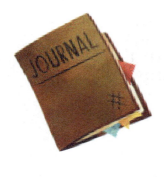

Journal prompts-Reflection and gratitude for today.

What made me smile today? What made me laugh? Who helped me? Who did I help? Who influenced me? How? Have I told them?

Who did I influence? How did I manage frustration/ disappointment? How did I honor God?

Is there anything I can improve?

_____

_____

_____

_____

"It is better to be content with what little you have. Otherwise, you will always be struggling for more. That is like chasing the wind." Ecclesiastes 4:6 (ICB)

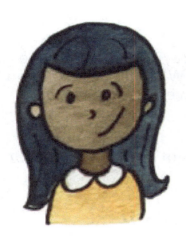

Draw or make a list of the people, places, and things for which you are grateful. Choose a person on your list and write them a letter of appreciation.

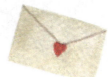

Hymn:
Count Your Blessings

How do you feel when you think about what you're grateful for? Let's say a prayer of thanks.

Dear God,

Thank you so much for _____. Please help me remember to be thankful in all circumstances just like you want me to be.

Using the letters of the alphabet, try to think of one thing you're grateful for per letter!

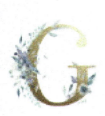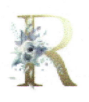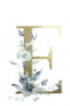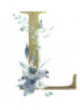

Contentment—Am I only happy when I get what I want? We will never get everything we want and we will always be left wanting more. This will lead to discontent and we will never be at peace. Can I appreciate what I have? This is where true contentment can be found. Write down a list of your blessings and thank God for what you have.

Read the following passage of Scripture and the context surrounding it. Do you know where Paul was when he wrote the book of Philippians? (Hint-it wasn't a very happy place!) Using this knowledge, how can you read this passage of Scripture with a new perspective on gratitude and contentment?

"I am very happy in the Lord that you have shown your care for me again. You continued to care about me, but there was no way for you to show it. I am telling you this, but it is not because I need anything. I have learned to be satisfied with the things I have and with everything that happens. I know how to live when I am poor. And I know how to live when I have plenty. I have learned the secret of being happy at any time in everything that happens. I have learned to be happy when I have enough to eat and when I do not have enough to eat. I have learned to be happy when I have all that I need and when I do not have the things I need. I can do all things through Christ because He gives me strength." Phil 4:10-13 (ICB)

WANTS   NEEDS

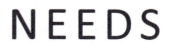

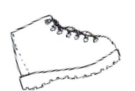

toys	God
electronics	food
name brand clothes	water
everything my friend has	shelter
name brand shoes	clothing
a big house	safety
to be "cool"	

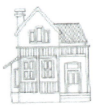

Is there anything you can add to this list?

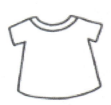

Read Exodus 16 together. Discuss how the Israelites were focused on what they were lacking rather than the blessings God had given them (and continued to give). Have you ever felt this way? Discuss with a loved one.

© Natalie Duhon

Take some time to write or draw your thoughts about this chapter.
Use the reflection questions on the next page to guide you!

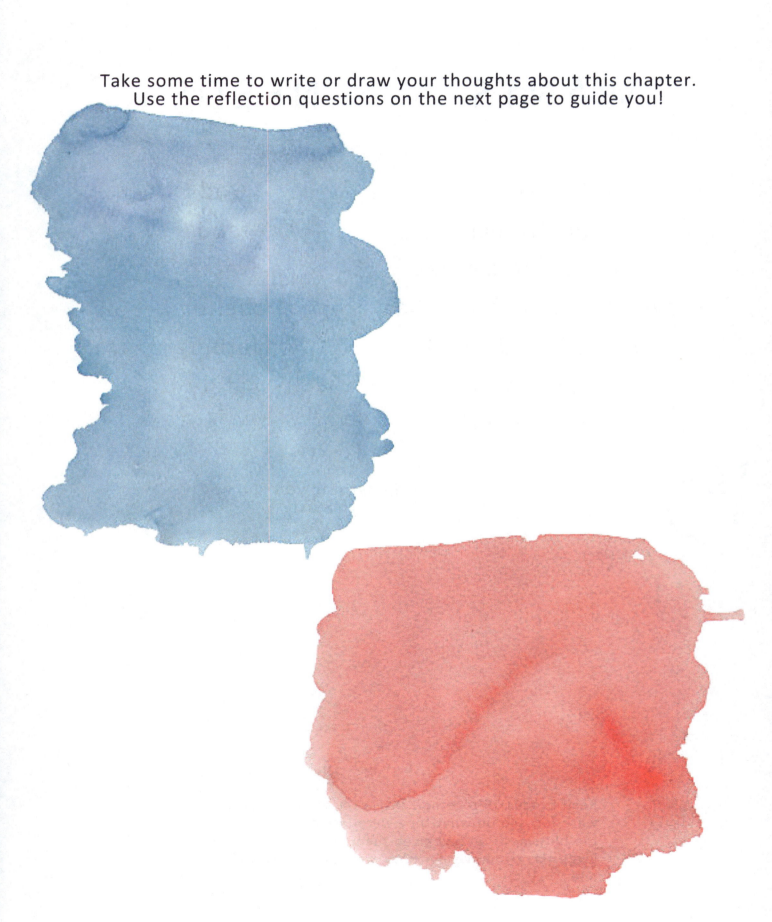

Reflection

What did you learn about gratitude, happiness, and peace?
How did this lesson add to the knowledge you already had?
What questions do you still have?
Name one thing you can do to begin doing to express gratitude. How will it impact your mood and your faith in God?
Look up the definitions of gratitude, happiness, and peace, and then find out what the Bible says. What are the similarities and differences?

Fun learning about emotions

Exercise 1: Create puppets to express different emotions. Use a brown paper bag to decorate it. Make one for happy, angry, worried, and sad. You can make more if you'd like! Use the puppets to practice expressing these emotions in a healthy way. Ask a loved one to help!

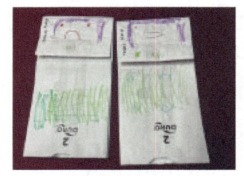

Elizabeth-age 7

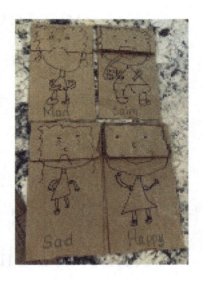

Camille-age 8

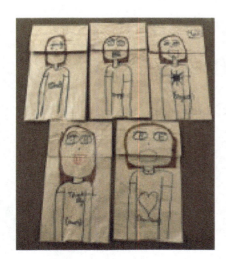

Audrey-age 10

Fun learning about emotions

Exercise 2: Create a calm down bag: fill it with things that help you calm down when you are worried, angry, or upset. Ideas include a Bible, prayer cards, headphones to listen to music, a stuffed animal, clay, a journal, drawing supplies, a soft blanket, a pretty picture, a sensory bag (instructions can be found online), coping cards, etc.

Exercise 3: Using age appropriate magazines, create a "feelings collage." Choose pictures that represent happy, sad, mad, and scared. You can add more feelings if you'd like.

Exercise 4: Using the list of emotions provided, create an index card for each emotion, along with their definition. (Practice using a dictionary by looking up the definition for each one). Have a loved one pick a card and you teach them or demonstrate what that emotion means!

Exercise 5: Watch your favorite movie or television show with a loved one and see if you can identify different emotions the characters experience. How did they handle them? Was it healthy/unhealthy? What could they have done differently?

Exercise 6: Keep an emotion log for one week. Write down how you feel during the day and what impacts your mood. Are there certain times of the day when you are more worried, mad, or sad? How about happy? Pay attention to your thoughts and behaviors. Also, pay attention to how your body feels. This will help improve your self-awareness. Remember, we all have emotions, and it's our job to control them! (See template and sample in appendix).

Exercise 7: On the outside of a lunch bag, draw how you appear on the outside. On the inside of the bag, draw how you really feel on the inside. Do they match? Do you ever try to hide how you're feeling? How can you express your emotions to a loved one?

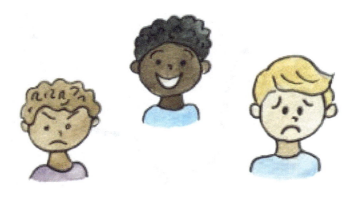

Exercise 8: Look up a picture of an iceberg. What makes an iceberg so significant is that the part of the iceberg you see above the water is only a small portion of the actual iceberg. The majority of it lies underneath the water. Picture your anger as the top of the iceberg. The giant piece of ice underneath the water represents all the extra emotions that are underneath your anger. Label them. (Examples might include resentment, sadness, guilt, worry, helplessness, etc.)

An example is located in the appendix.

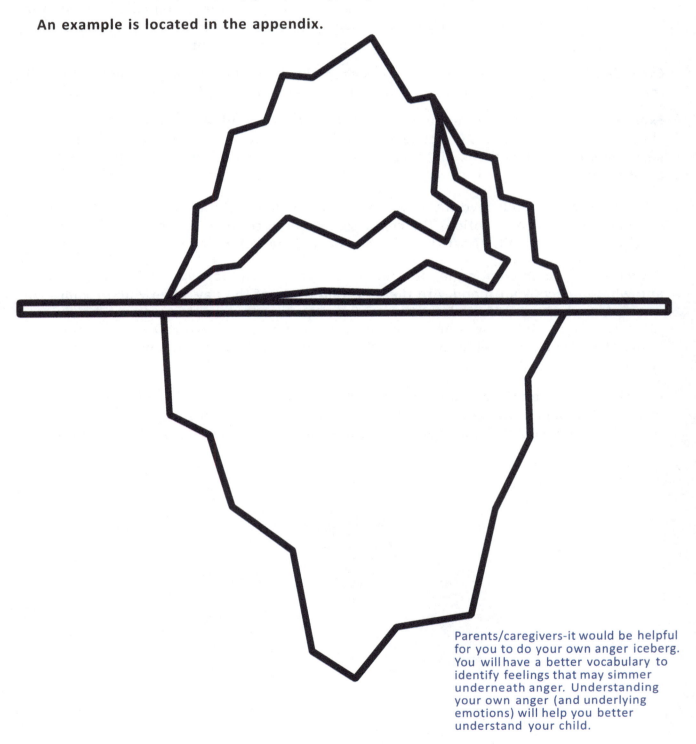

Parents/caregivers-it would be helpful for you to do your own anger iceberg. You will have a better vocabulary to identify feelings that may simmer underneath anger. Understanding your own anger (and underlying emotions) will help you better understand your child.

Exercise 9: Using blank index cards, create coping flash cards. On each card, write down a helpful coping skill and on the other side, draw a picture of that coping skill. Or, with an adult's help, you can print a picture of that coping skill. You can also make copies of the pictures in this book.

Exercise 10: Do a body scan. Pay attention to each part of your body, starting from the top of your head, all the way down to your toes. Where do you feel tension/tightness? Where do you feel relaxed? Our mental and physical health are intricately connected, so it's very helpful to pay attention to what our body is trying to tell us.

Exercise 11: The next time you feel stressed, angry, or sad, pay attention to what you notice about your behavior. Ask a trusted adult about what they noticed. The better we get at identifying how we think, feel, and act when we are upset, the more effective we will be at learning to manage these feelings.

Exercise 12: Pick your favorite coloring page or activity page from the back of this book. You can also choose one you already have. Notice how you feel while coloring or completing a fun activity. How does it help? You can also play relaxing music during this exercise.

Exercise 13: Play! All of us, especially children, need to do things that are fun and bring us joy. This can improve how we feel and our relationship with others. Take some time to do something fun together. This can be a game, sports, or a fun competition. Be creative!

Exercise 14: Utilize the skill of guided imagery. Guided imagery involves imagining a peaceful scene to help you relax. How many of your five senses can you use? Frequently used scenes include a beach, a meadow, the mountains, or a forest. There are many apps and videos that are beneficial. Another helpful skill is progressive muscle relaxation, which guides you to tense and relax various muscle groups. There are numerous resources for both of these skills, as well as adaptations for young children. I recommend you screen them first, to ensure they align with your Christian beliefs.

Exercise 15: Play a game of charades! This game is great to improve communication skills and awareness of emotions.

Exercise 16: Look in the mirror and demonstrate different emotions. Use your emotion cards!

Exercise 17: Everyone likes using baking soda and vinegar to make a volcano. Find instructions online for how to make a homemade volcano and talk about the anger analogy we discussed earlier! It's a great visual and a helpful way to explore how our anger might cause us to explode like a volcano.

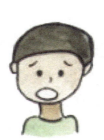
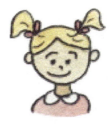
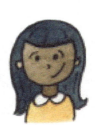

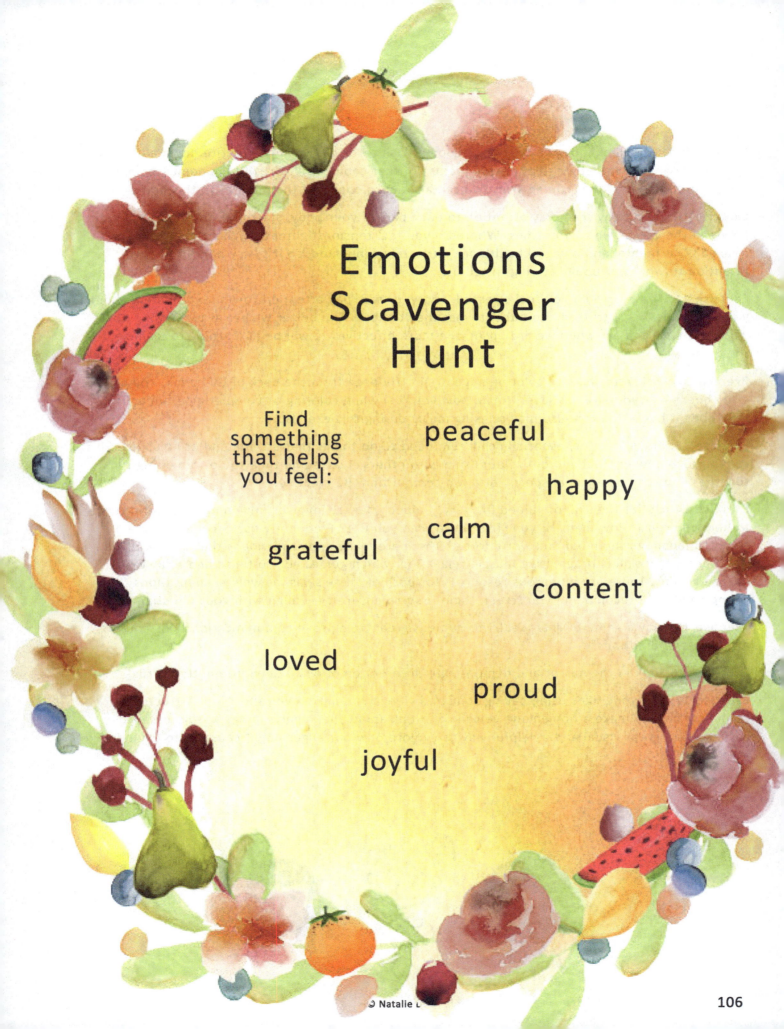

Emotions Scavenger Hunt

Find something that helps you feel:

peaceful

happy

calm

grateful

content

loved

proud

joyful

Let's see what you've learned about emotions! Match each behavior/physical sensation to an emotion. Some may fit into more than one category.

Anxiety

Love

Anger

Happiness

Sadness

empathy
crying
muscle tension
irritability
caring
arguing/yelling
catastrophizing
smiling
difficulty concentrating
kindness
negative thinking
sleep disturbance
fast heart beat
shaking
laughing
blaming
upset stomach
spending time together
loss of interest
avoidance
being helpful
ruminating

Words to know: **Catastrophizing** is when we make a problem seem worse than it really is. We worry about the worst possible outcome and focus on that. **Ruminating** is when we think about the same thing over and over like a broken record. The only thing we should ruminate on is the word of God!

Take some time to write or draw your thoughts about this chapter.
Use the reflection questions on the next page to guide you!

Reflection

What did you learn about your emotions after completing some of the previous exercises?
Which one was most helpful?
Pick one or two of these exercises to practice regularly. This will help you learn healthier ways to identify and manage your emotions!
Can you think of your own?

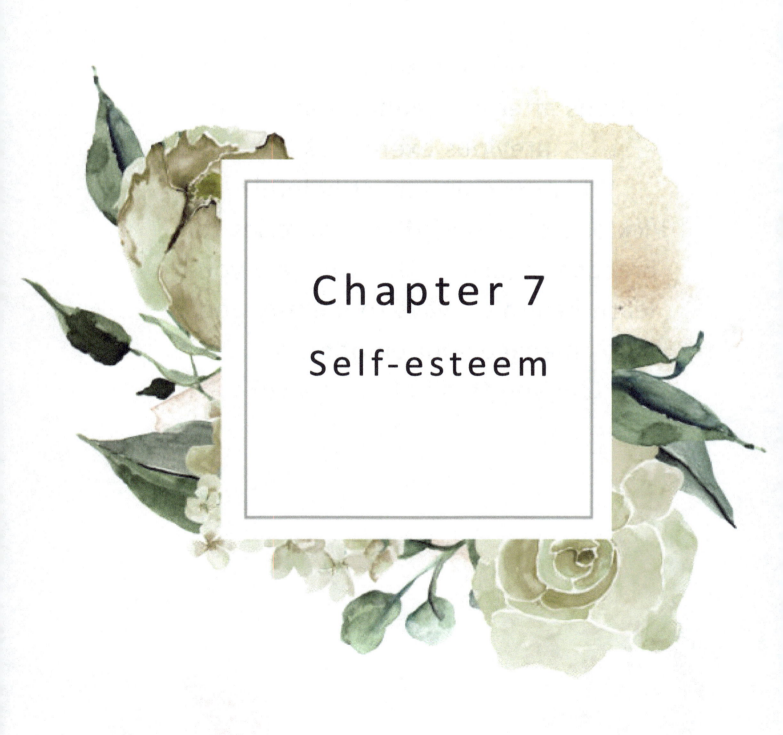

Chapter 7
Self-esteem

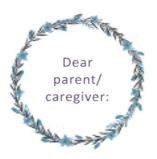

Dear parent/caregiver:

Our children (and ourselves) are constantly bombarded with society's view of self-worth. Who and what are they watching/listening to? What messages are they hearing about their appearance and self-worth? How does it compare to what the Bible tells us?

What do they hear you say about your looks, weight, etc.? What do they hear you say about others? How does gossip affect our self-esteem? How are our children impacted when we gossip about others? What does the Bible say about gossip?

As parents/caregivers, we are our children's first role models. If we constantly criticize them or they hear us criticize ourselves, those will become our child's learned thoughts and behaviors. Our self-talk will become their self-talk. Are we affirming them as made in God's image? Are we affirming ourselves as made in God's image?

Parent/caregiver journal: Self-esteem is a huge issue, especially for women. Take some time to journal your thoughts about your own self-esteem and self-worth. What factors in your life have played a role in how you feel about yourself? We tend to be our harshest critics. Take some time to explore these feelings and share with a therapist or a loved one.

Self-esteem is how we feel or think about ourselves. We often determine self-esteem by our looks, the clothes we wear, the car we drive, how much money we have, the house we live in, and how smart we are. What does the Bible say? Look up some Bible verses about self-esteem and write about what you learned.

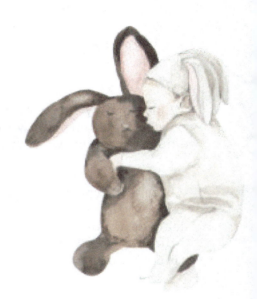

Psalm 139:13-16 (ICB) tells us: **"You made my whole being. You formed me in my mother's body. I praise you because you made me in an amazing and wonderful way. What you have done is wonderful. I know this very well. You saw my bones being formed as I took shape in my mother's body. When I was put together there, you saw my body as it was formed. All the days planned for me were written in your book before I was one day old."**

Self-esteem

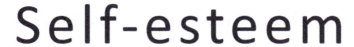

I was created for relationship with my heavenly Father. He knows every hair on my head. God created me to love me and so I can love Him.

Exercise 1-Write a letter to yourself describing how God feels about you (Use direct quotes from the Bible).

Exercise 2-Ask a loved one to write a letter to you describing how much they love you and why.

Exercise 3-Draw a picture of yourself the way God sees you. What makes you beautiful to God? (kind, loving, helpful, patient, etc.)

Exercise 4-Jesus died for us. There is no greater love than His! Journal your thoughts about this profound truth.

Exercise 5-Parents/caregivers-ask several of your child's loved ones to write them a short note of affirmation. Help them make a journal or scrapbook with these notes. They will treasure it forever. (Add your favorite Bible verses to speak truth to your child).

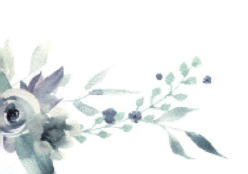

"God has made us what we are. In Christ Jesus, God made us new people so that we would do good works. God had planned in advance those good works for us. He had planned for us to live our lives doing them." Ephesians 2:10 (ICB)

What does the Bible say about beauty?

"It is not fancy hair, gold jewelry, or fine clothes that should make you beautiful. No, your beauty should come from within you—the beauty of a gentle and quiet spirit. This beauty will never disappear, and it is worth very much to God." 1 Pet 3:3-4 (ICB)

"Charm can fool you, and beauty can trick you. But a woman who respects the Lord should be praised." Proverbs 31:30 (ICB)

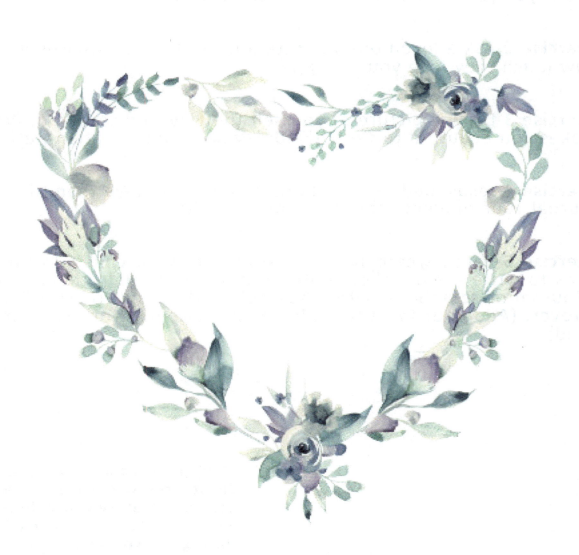

Using your Bible, write down some ways God sees you.

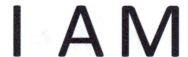

I AM

free	John 8:36
a child of God	1 John 3:1
chosen	Mark 13:27
loved	John 3:16
right in His sight	Rom. 3:24
bold	Heb. 4:16
comforted	2 Cor. 1:3-4
strong	Eph. 6:10
forgiven	Matt. 6:14
a good work	Phil. 1:6
God's masterpiece	Eph. 2:10
redeemed	Gal. 3:13
valuable	Matt. 10:31
encouraged	Acts 20:2
forgiven	Eph. 4:32
able	Eph. 6:11

Pick one of these verses to memorize and remind yourself who you are in Christ. Write it down and place it where you will see it often. Ask a trusted family member or friend to speak this truth into your life often.

How do these truths differ from what the world tells us?

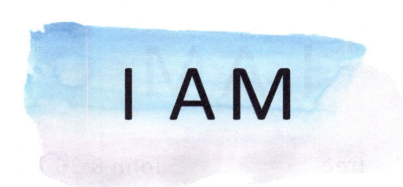

I AM

```
H S E C H O S E N C H M T D J L E D W F
V G I L S T F U O L I L H P E M N K I G
P M U I H B C X L P O I U T E G H V J V
M A L V G S T R O N G C R E H C E V L P
M S O H V R G B V N C N D O L H F A V R
O T K H V R T H E N K E I N J Y R L V B
L E N Y H J V F D F R V J V F T Y U A R
I R M O L H F R Y H N I O P L I G A B F
M P H B N F C F H J L G P L I H Y B T Y
M I B B O L D N J D D R K L O H B L V T
M E B H Y I K F X S C O M F O R T E D P
M C M L H M V D H T D F H B T I L O P B
G E K K S H L P J G V B M I U Y G F D L
M I Y H N G V D F R A B L E L P O H B Y
```

COMFORTED   STRONG

FORGIVEN   MASTERPIECE

BOLD   CHOSEN

VALUABLE   ABLE

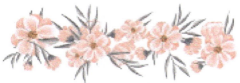

Write or draw some of your strengths. Then ask a few loved ones to help you add to the list. (Examples include: caring, kind, friendly, loving, patient, determined, etc.). How can you use these strengths to help yourself and others?

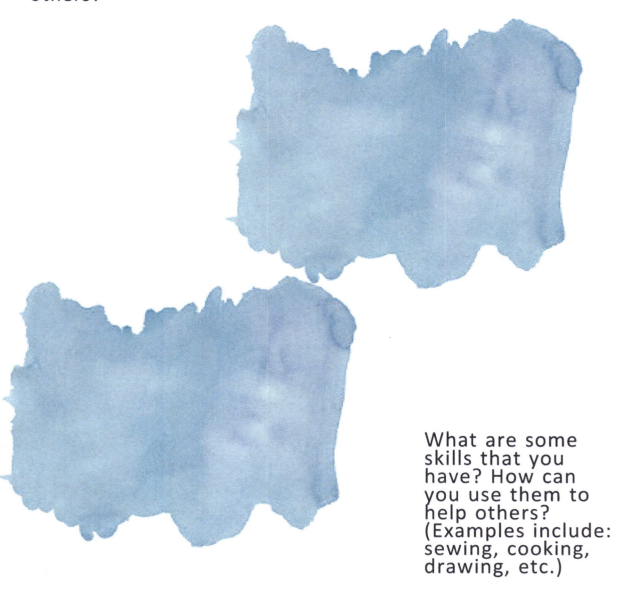

What are some skills that you have? How can you use them to help others? (Examples include: sewing, cooking, drawing, etc.)

Listen to the hymn "Do You Know That You Were Chosen"

Draw your thoughts and feelings about God's love for you as you listen.

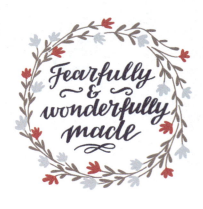

Using an ink pad, create your own fingerprint. When God created you, He gave you your own fingerprint. No one else has it! Use a magnifying glass to see your fingerprint up close. Write a prayer of thanks to God for making you unique. Remember that God created every person for a purpose!

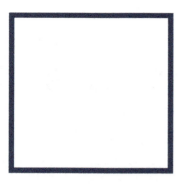

My unique fingerprint!

Hymn: I Stand Amazed (O How Marvelous)

_____

_____

_____

_____

Take some time to write or draw your thoughts about this chapter.
Use the reflection questions on the next page to guide you!

Reflection

What did you learn about self-esteem? How did this lesson add to the knowledge you already had about self-esteem?
What questions do you still have?
Name one thing you can do to begin finding your worth in God.
Look up the definition of self-esteem, then find out what the Bible says. What are the similarities and differences?
Which self-esteem exercise was the most impactful?

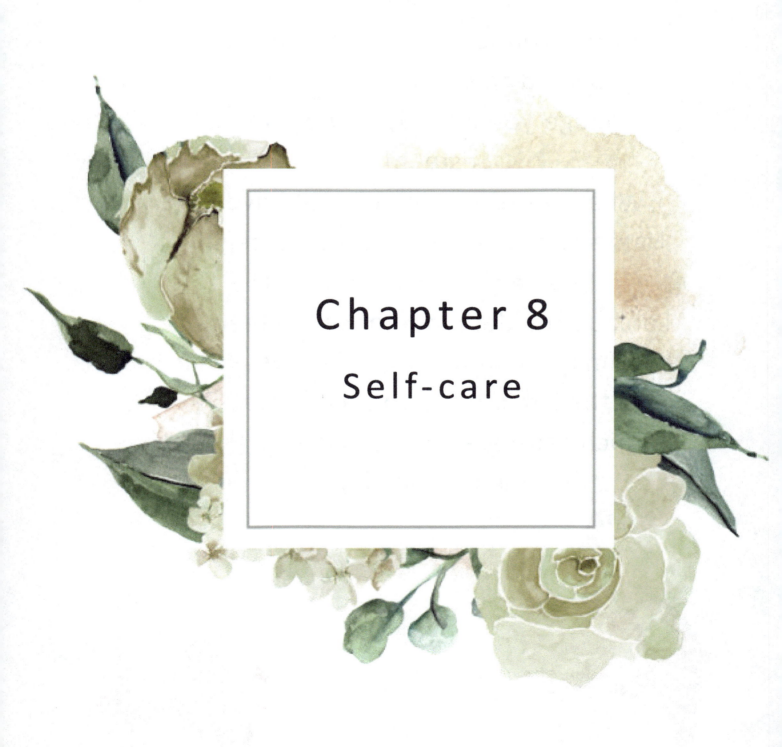

Chapter 8
Self-care

It's hard to be calm when I don't feel well. I need to check in with my physical, spiritual, and mental health. Here are some simple questions I can keep in mind that will help me determine how I'm feeling and what I can do about it. Is there something on my mind that I'm feeling sad about? Worried? Confused? Do I have other feelings underneath my anger? (embarrassed, jealous, resentful, bored).

Am I spending too much time worrying about something? Am I holding on to a grudge? Have I spent time with other people who love me or have I felt a little lonely? Are they encouraging and supporting me? Are they helping hold me accountable?

Have I been spending time reading God's word and talking to Him through prayer? Write down your thoughts here.

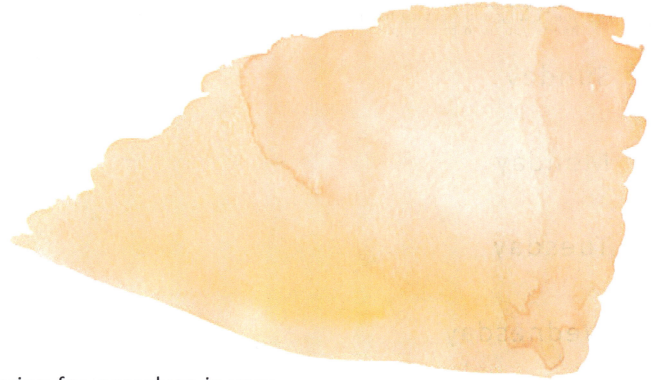

Caring for ourselves is very important. It's hard to serve God and other people if we aren't taking care of our basic needs.

God didn't need to rest on the last day of creation week. He did it to set the pattern for us. God has instructed us to care for all aspects of ourselves. Keeping a log of the following aspects of self-care can help us determine which factors impact our mental health.

Am I hungry?
Did I get enough sleep?
Did I eat too much sugar?
Am I getting ill?

Am I tired?
Did I drink enough water?
Have I gotten any exercise?

Sometimes what we eat or drink can have an impact on our mood. How do you feel when you consume too much sugar, fat, or caffeine? How do you feel when you don't get enough exercise or time outdoors? How does your mood change when you don't get enough sleep? Try keeping a journal of your eating and sleeping habits for the next week or two. Are there any habits you need to change?

Sunday

Monday

Tuesday

Wednesday

Thursday

Friday

Saturday

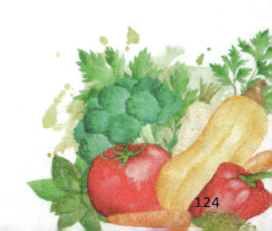

Circle the foods that are healthy to eat. What we eat can impact our mood, so try to eat as many healthy foods as you can!

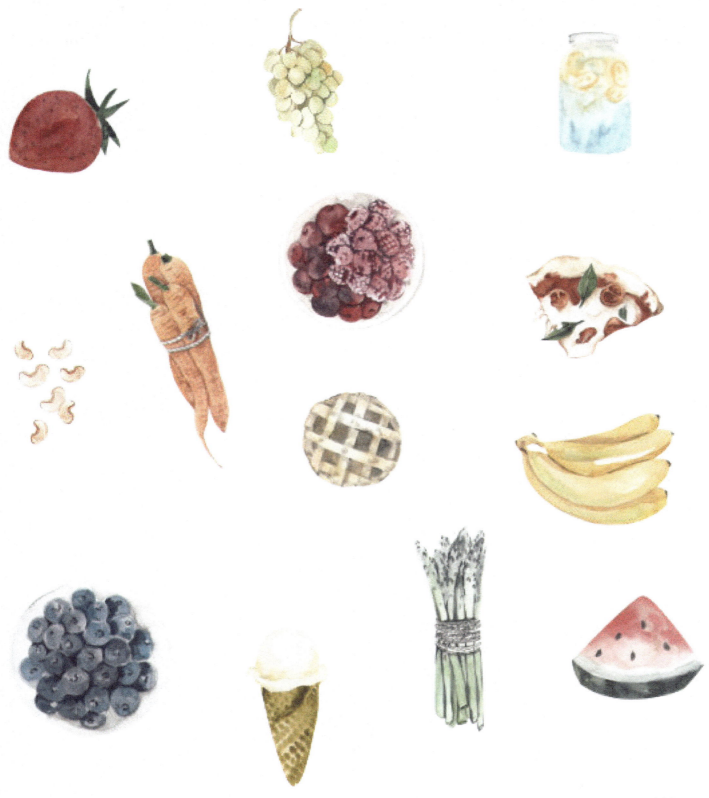

Caring for our hygiene is important. Hygiene is a fancy word for making sure we are taking care of our bodies. This includes brushing and flossing our teeth, washing our hair and body, and wearing clean clothes. It also includes things such as clipping our nails and making sure we wash our hands regularly. This helps us feel better about ourselves and helps prevent us from getting sick!

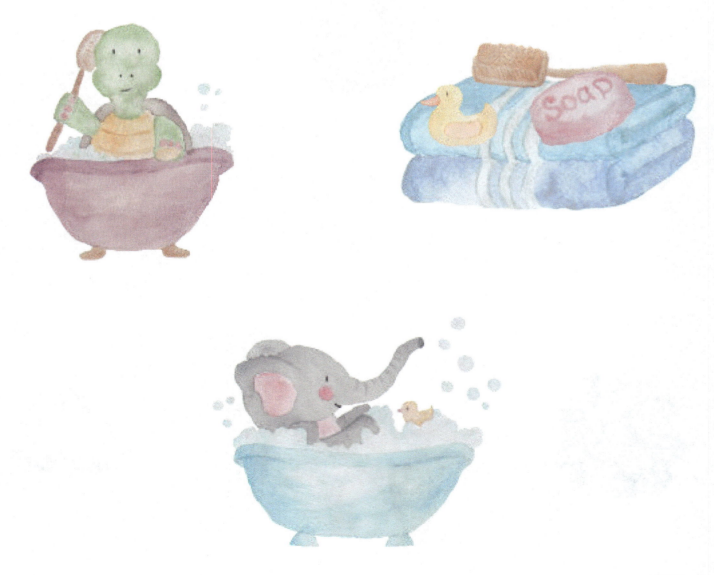

Take some time to write or draw your thoughts about this chapter.
Use the reflection questions on the next page to guide you!

Reflection

What did you learn about self-care and hygiene?

How did this lesson add to the knowledge you already had about self-care and hygiene?

What questions do you still have?

Name one thing you can do to improve your self-care.

What does the Bible say about caring for yourself? This includes our physical body as well as our spiritual and mental well-being.

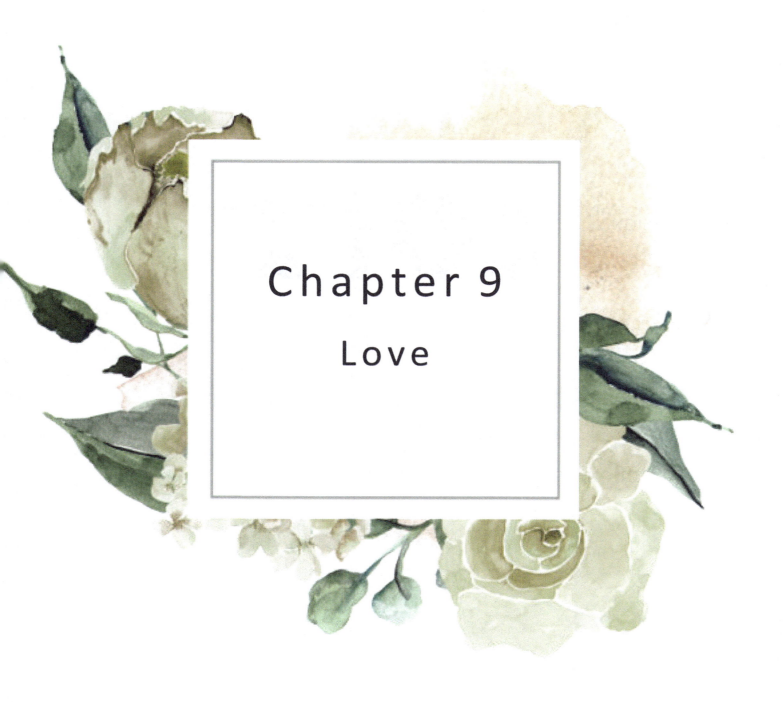

Chapter 9
Love

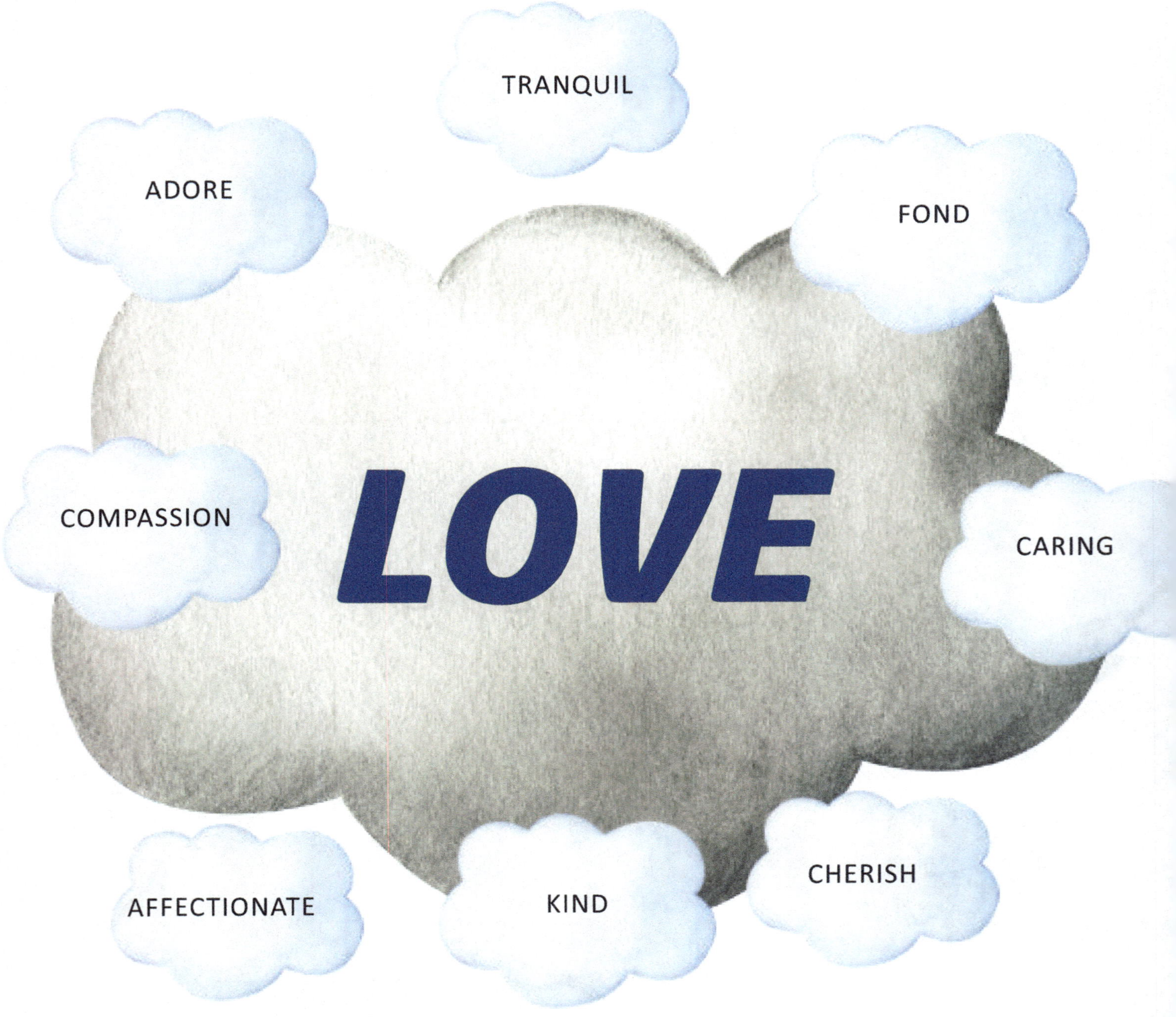

LOVE

- TRANQUIL
- ADORE
- FOND
- COMPASSION
- CARING
- AFFECTIONATE
- KIND
- CHERISH

"I may speak in different languages of men or even angels. But if I do not have love, then I am only a noisy bell or a ringing cymbal. I may have the gift of prophecy; I may understand all the secret things of God and all knowledge; and I may have faith so great that I can move mountains. But even with all these things, if I do not have love, then I am nothing. I may give everything I have to feed the poor. And I may even give my body as an offering to be burned. But I gain nothing by doing these things if I do not have love. Love is patient and kind. Love is not jealous, it does not brag, and it is not proud. Love is not rude, is not selfish, and does not become angry easily. Love does not remember wrongs done against it. Love takes no pleasure in evil, but rejoices over the truth. Love patiently accepts all things. It always trusts, always hopes, and always continues strong."

1 Cor 13:1-7 (ICB)

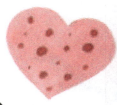

How can I love others?

In the Bible, we learn that we all descended from Adam and Eve. This means we were created in the image of God. Unfortunately, there are many people that judge others and are mean to them based on what they look like. This could be the color of their skin, differences in eye or hair color, or how they sound. They may also judge others based on their different abilities (wheelchair, prosthetic arm/leg). Some people may have hidden disabilities that we aren't even aware of. Some people are judged because of their culture or because their behavior doesn't look like ours. We need to remember that every person we will ever meet is created by and loved by God. We should treat others with kindness. We can recognize, accept, and celebrate each others' differences!

"This is how we know what real love is: Jesus gave His life for us. So we should give our lives for our brothers. Suppose a believer is rich enough to have all that he needs. He sees his brother in Christ who is poor and does not have what he needs. What if the believer does not help the poor brother? Then the believer does not have God's love in his heart." 1 John 3:16-17 (ICB)

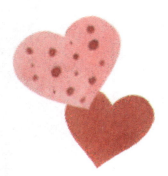

Today's activity will be borrowing a book from the library about a group of people who might look different from you. What can you learn about them? How are you similar? Remind yourself that they were made by God just like you are!

"God began by making one man. From him came all the different people who live everywhere in the world. He decided exactly when and where they must live." Acts 17:26 (ICB)

"If you make fun of the poor, you insult God, who made them." Proverbs 17:5 (ICB)

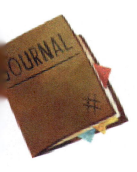

Journal your thoughts about loving others who look different than you. What did you learn from your book from the library? How can you continue to learn about others and practice loving them? Write a prayer asking God to help you love others just as He loves us.

"For God loved the world so much that He gave His only Son. God gave His Son so that whoever believes in Him may not be lost, but have eternal life." John 3:16 (ICB)

_____

_____

_____

_____

"Your love must be real. Hate what is evil. Hold on to what is good. Love each other like brothers and sisters. Give your brothers and sisters more honor than you want for yourselves." Romans 12:9-10 (ICB)

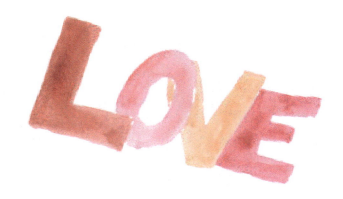

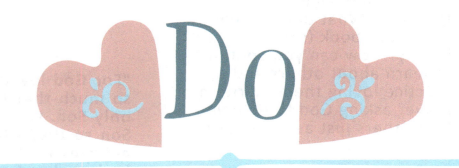
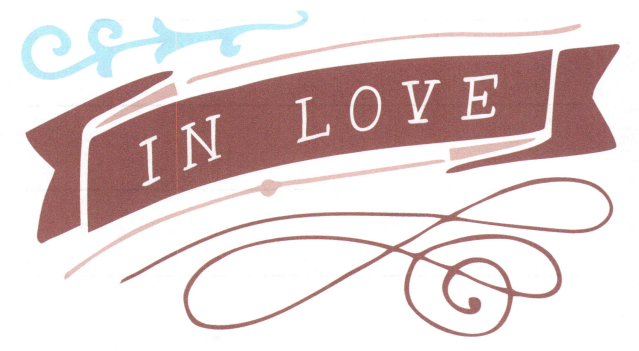

How can I serve others? What does the Bible say about serving?

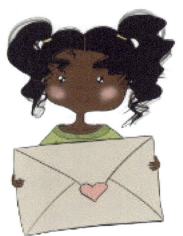

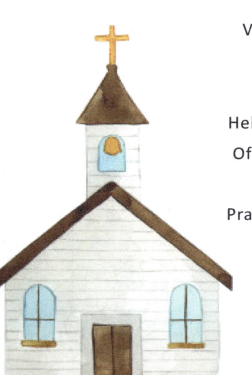

Write a card/letter
Volunteer at church
Bake something
Cook a meal
Help clean their house
Offer encouragement
Call them
Pray for them and with them
Help them with yard work
Plant a garden
Visit them
Open the door for them
Carry their groceries
Make them a gift (sew, color, paint)
Take their trash out
Volunteer at an animal shelter
Visit someone in the hospital
Visit someone in the nursing home
Clean up litter

"Do your work, and be happy to do it. Work as if you were serving the Lord, not as if you were serving only men."
Ephesians 6:7 (ICB)

Choose one way you can serve someone else. Draw yourself serving here and ask your parent/caregiver for a way you can make it happen in your church or community! How does serving help improve your mood?

"Each of you received a spiritual gift. God has shown you His grace in giving you different gifts. And you are like servants who are responsible for using God's gifts. So be good servants and use your gifts to serve each other."
1 Peter 4:10 (ICB)

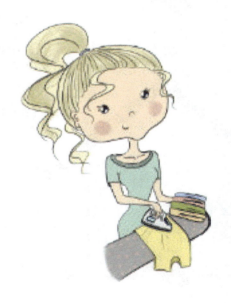

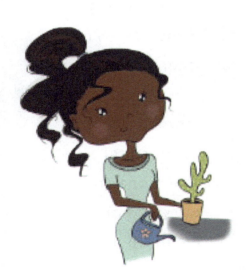

"In all the work you are doing, work the best you can. Work as if you were working for the Lord, not for men."
Colossians 3:23 (ICB)

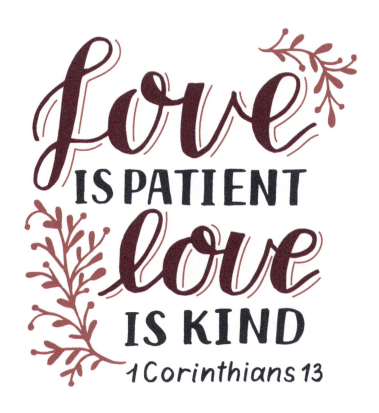

What does it mean to be patient and kind? How do these traits help us love others? How does being loving, kind, and patient impact our mental health?

Take some time to write or draw your thoughts about this chapter. Use the reflection questions on the next page to guide you!

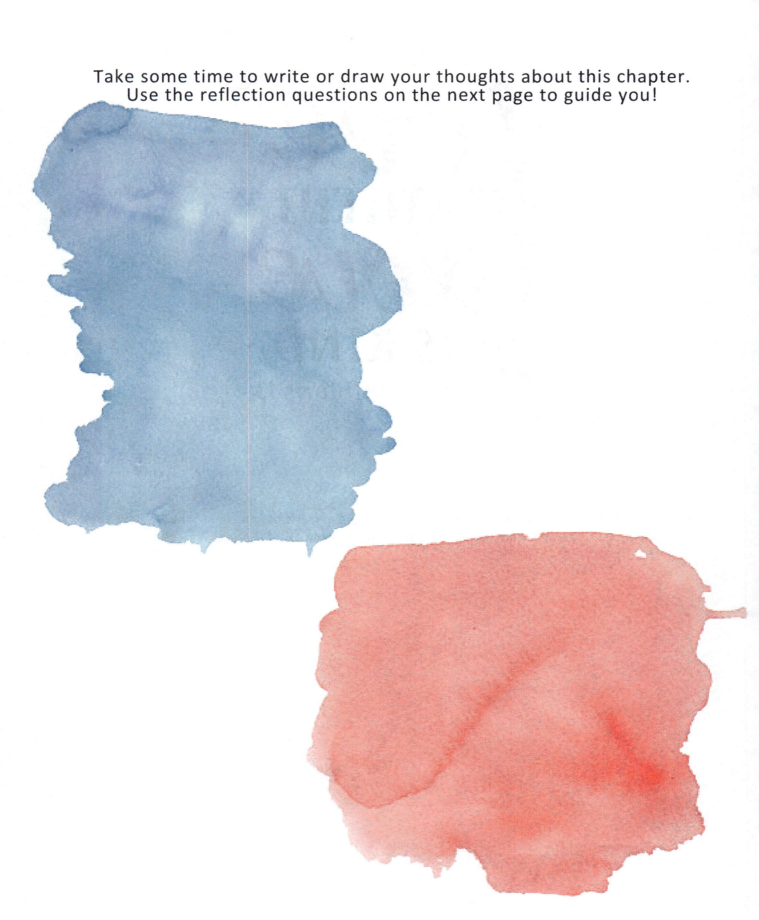

Reflection

What did you learn about love? How did this lesson add to the knowledge you already had? What questions do you still have? Name one thing you can do to begin doing to express love for God, others, and yourself.
Look up the definition of love and then find out what the Bible says. What are the similarities and differences?
"For God so loved the world that He gave His only Son." John 3:16 (ICB)
What does the word love mean to you after reading this passage of Scripture?

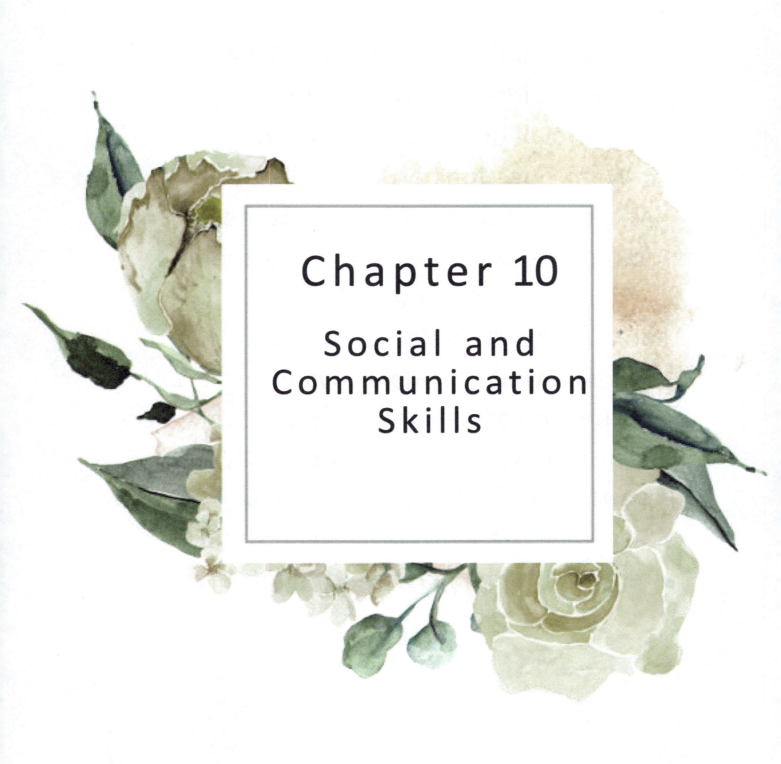

Chapter 10

Social and Communication Skills

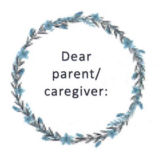

Dear parent/caregiver:

Social skills are an important part of being able to function in society. Although we ultimately answer to God, it is beneficial for us to learn about, and model appropriate social and communication skills for our children. We teach these best by serving as role models for our children. What can we learn from the Bible about how we should interact with and treat others? How do you model social skills for your child? Children need specific instructions on how to communicate well and they need opportunities to practice.

Parent/caregiver journal: What were you taught about social skills? Did you learn by observing or did you parents teach you specific rules to follow? Who modeled good communication for you? Do you find it easy to socialize with others or more difficult?

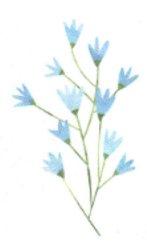

What does the Bible say about how we should treat others?

Am I living to please others or to please God?

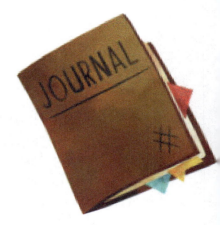

Luke 6:37 (ICB) says: **"Don't judge other people, and you will not be judged. Don't accuse others of being guilty, and you will not be accused of being guilty. Forgive other people, and you will be forgiven."**

"Brothers, someone in your group might do something wrong. You who are spiritual should go to him and help make him right again. You should do this in a gentle way. But be careful! You might be tempted to sin, too. Help each other with your troubles. When you do this, you truly obey the law of Christ." Galatians 6:1-2 (ICB)

Journal your thoughts on these verses:

_____

_____

_____

_____

Communication Skills

Eye contact-Make eye contact with the other person, but don't stare. Let the other person know you're listening to them.

Listening skills-if you focus more on your response, you'll miss what the other person is saying. Active listening is when you really try to understand what the other person is saying. It's harder than you think!

Words-Are your words helpful or hurtful? Remember, the person you are talking to is a child of God just like you are. Do your words honor God?

Voice-Are you talking too loud/soft? Fast/slow? What is your tone? What emotions are you conveying? Do you have trouble clearly articulating your thoughts? (These all take practice!)

Questions-Are you asking questions to clarify what the person is telling you?

Do you interrupt or **wait** for the other person to finish speaking?

Do you assume you know what the other person is thinking?

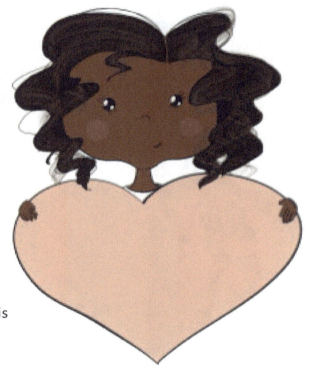

Do you need to **calm down**/take a break before having a difficult conversation? Do you need to ask a trusted adult for help communicating?

Do you demand that you always get what you want without considering the other person's needs?

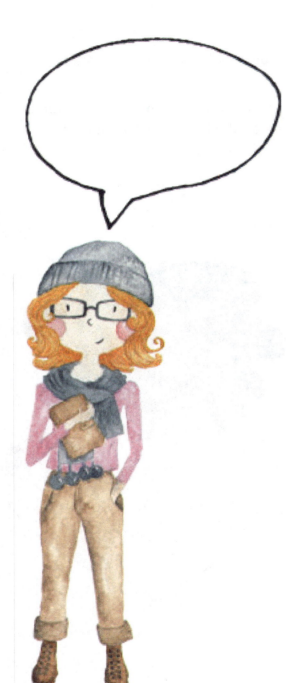

A significant amount of our communication is **nonverbal**. This means we communicate without words. This includes body language, posture, and **eye contact**.

What do you communicate with your **body language**? What about **hand gestures** or other body movement? Do you nod your head to communicate you understand what the other person is saying? Are you fidgeting or restless? Can you try your best to stay still and listen to the other person?

How's your **facial expression**? Are you making mean faces? Are you rolling your eyes? Does your facial expression show that you are interested in what the other person is trying to say? Are you smiling? Do you look confused?

Boundaries-Are you too far from or close to the person you are speaking to?

Posture-Are you facing the person? Are you nodding to indicate you are listening? Are you sitting up ready to listen, or slouched over with a bored look on your face?

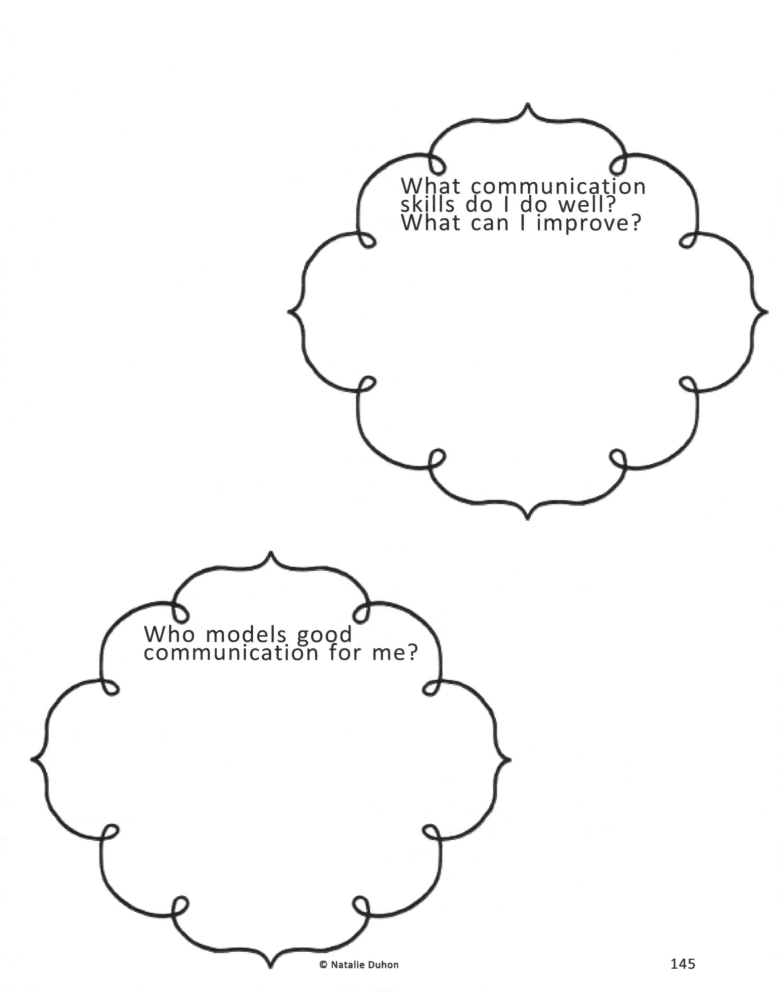

Let's practice our listening skills!

Exercise 1

Have a loved one read a passage of Scripture. Be sure to listen closely! Then tell it back in your own words.

Exercise 2

Have a loved on read a poem or short story to you. Do your best to listen to what is being said. Then tell it back in your own words. (You can also draw a picture).

Exercise 3

Have a loved one pretend not to listen to you when you are speaking to them. How do you feel? How might someone else feel when you don't listen to them?

Exercise 4

Play a game of Simon Says or Telephone! How do these games help improve our listening skills?

Exercise 5

Have a loved one describe a picture for you to draw. (Nothing too difficult). Is it easy or hard to follow their directions? Example: Draw a house with two windows and one door. Color the door blue. Draw two pink flowers in the yard, etc.

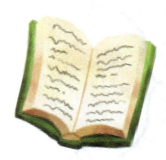

Reminder: Don't get so caught up in the next thing you want to say that you forget to listen to what the other person is telling you!

© Natalie Duhon

Let's practice your social skills!

What areas of your life can you practice using social skills?

Order food at a restaurant.
Speak to the cashier at a store.
Call a business on the phone.
Call family/friends on the phone.
Schedule an appointment.
Introduce yourself to a new friend.
Ask a worker a question at the store.

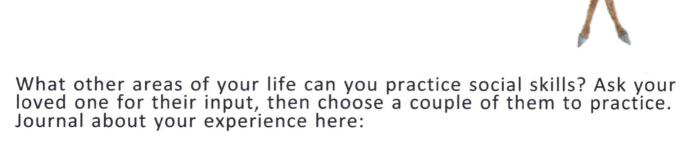

What other areas of your life can you practice social skills? Ask your loved one for their input, then choose a couple of them to practice. Journal about your experience here:

_____

_____

_____

_____

Communication Styles

<u>Aggressive</u>-getting what you want/need without caring about the other person's feelings and what they need

<u>Passive</u>-not getting what you want/need because you are afraid to speak up

<u>Assertive</u>-getting what you want/need while also respecting the other person and what they want/need

Example: A friend takes your favorite toy
Aggressive-Hit, kick, scream, grab the toy out of their hand
Passive-Do nothing, but feel very upset about the situation
Assertive-Calmly tell your friend that it is your favorite toy and ask them to return it

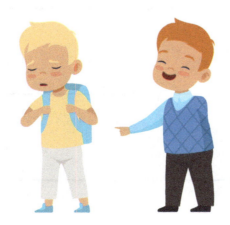

There are common behaviors associated with each communication style. Let's explore them in more depth.

Aggressive

1. May use sarcasm.
2. May interrupt and be disrespectful.
3. Tone of voice is harsh and loud.
4. Sees other people as less important.
5. Intimidating posture and intense stare.
6. Angry
7. Unwilling to compromise.
8. Does not respect another person's boundaries.

Assertive

1. Polite and firm.
2. Makes appropriate eye contact.
3. All persons involved are worthy of respect.
4. Friendly
5. Willing to compromise.
6. Able to set boundaries and respect the boundaries of others.
7. Tone of voice is pleasant.

Passive

1. Submissive and compliant.
2. Afraid to voice opinion or needs.
3. May avoid eye contact.
4. Restless, nervous behavior.
5. Gives in easily.
6. Unable to set boundaries.
7. Speaks very quietly.

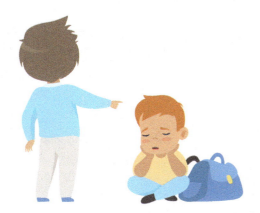

Can you think of examples of times when you demonstrated each of these communication styles? How do other people feel when we communicate in an aggressive manner?

What are some ways you can improve your ability to be assertive? Write down some ways here. (Remember, it takes practice).

Take a moment to pray and ask God to help you improve the way you communicate with others.

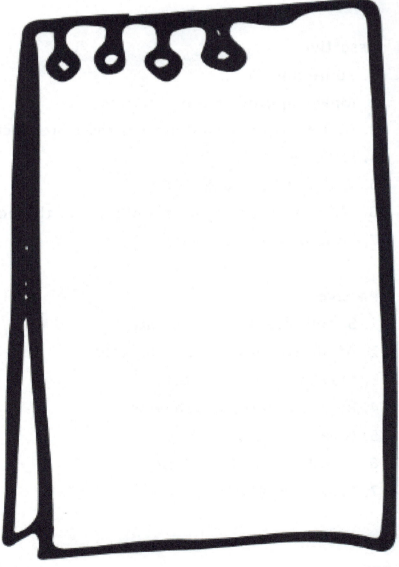

If someone is ever acting aggressive or you feel unsafe, be sure to ask a trusted adult for help.

Let's practice identifying different types of communication.

Read the following examples and see if you can determine which communication style was demonstrated. (Assertive, aggressive, passive).

Matthew was waiting in line and Caleb cut in front of him. Matthew politely told him, "Excuse me, I was next in line."

Susie was watching her favorite show on TV and her brother changed the channel. Susie started yelling at him and calling him names.

Elizabeth and Candace were playing with their dolls and Elizabeth took Candace's doll. Candace wanted to say something, but didn't because she was afraid of how Elizabeth would react.

Nicole and Charlie were waiting in line and Jack cut in front of them. Charlie pushed him out of the way and said loudly, "I was here first!"

Elizabeth did not want to hug her cousins when they came to visit. Instead of being rude, she was firm and direct, stating, "I do not want to hug you right now. Please respect my personal space."

Discuss these examples and how the response was appropriate or inappropriate. What could these children have done differently?

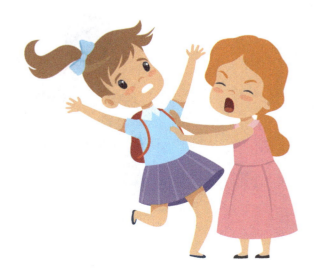

1. assertive
2. aggressive
3. passive
4. aggressive
5. assertive

Look at the following pictures. Take some time to discuss what is happening and how these children can behave differently.

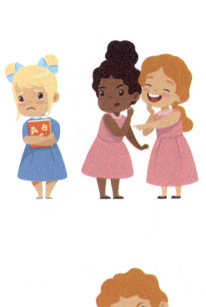
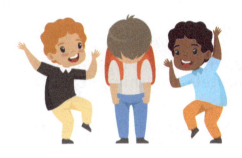
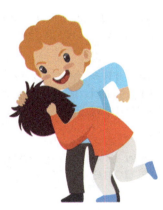
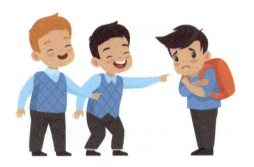
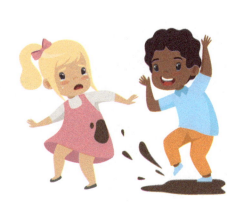
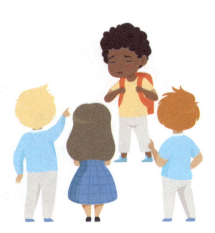

Can you think of behaviors that would hinder our communication with others? (To hinder means to make something worse). Brainstorm some ideas here and then we will discuss them on the next page.

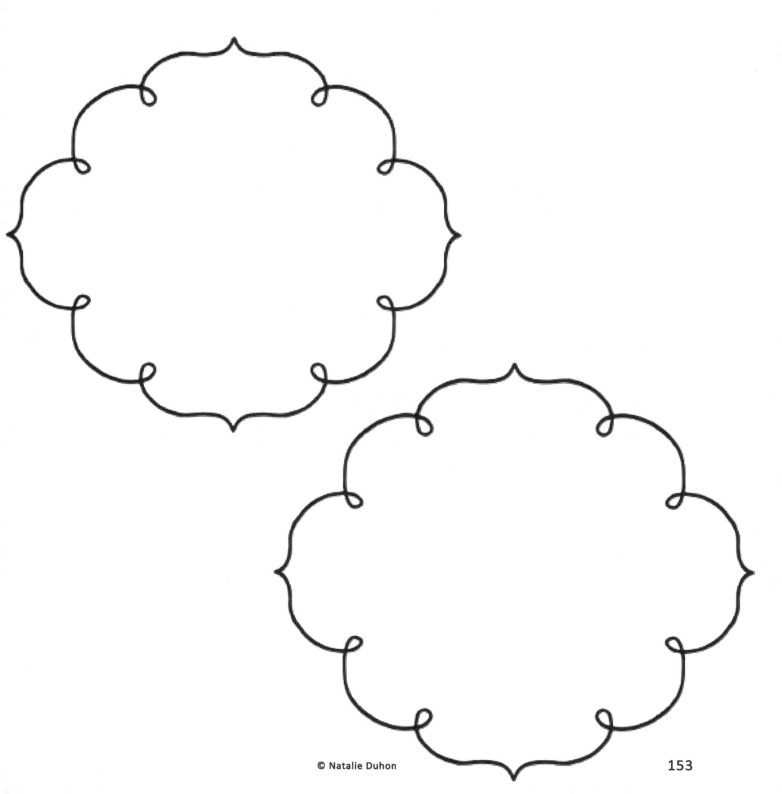

Barriers to communication

1. Blaming our behavior on someone else.
2. Demanding someone else do what we want.
3. Threatening behavior (this is never okay!)
4. Arguing
5. Judging
6. Name calling
7. Making excuses for our behavior.
8. Teasing
9. Sarcasm
10. Avoiding responsibility for our thoughts/actions.
11. Silent treatment

Remember the golden rule?
Treat others how we want to be treated!
Write the golden rule here.

_____

_____

_____

What have you learned so far about communication? Take some time to draw a picture demonstrating each style of communication. Talk about how you would describe each one and give examples. (Aggressive, assertive, passive)

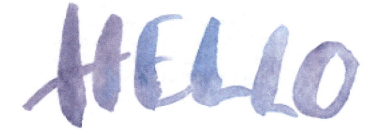

Even if we dislike someone, we still need to treat them with kindness and respect. Remember, no matter how someone acts, they are made in the image of God. Another person's behavior does not control yours. You are the only person who is in control of your behavior and how you treat others. We may not know what another person is going through and why they act the way they do. God always wants us to choose kindness and forgiveness.

"But God has wisdom and power. He has good advice and understanding." Job 12:13 (ICB)

"We must not become tired of doing good. We will receive our harvest of eternal life at the right time. We must not give up! When we have the opportunity to help anyone, we should do it. But we should give special attention to those who are in the family of believers." Galatians 6:9-10 (ICB)

Remember, since we are human, it's inevitable that we will make mistakes. We can apologize to the other person and ask for their forgiveness. We can ask God for His forgiveness and ask Him to help us do better next time.

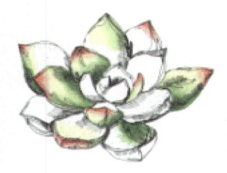

Genesis 1:27 (ICB) tells us "So God created human beings in His image. In the image of God He created them. He created them male and female."

Take some time to write or draw your thoughts about this chapter.
Use the reflection questions on the next page to guide you!

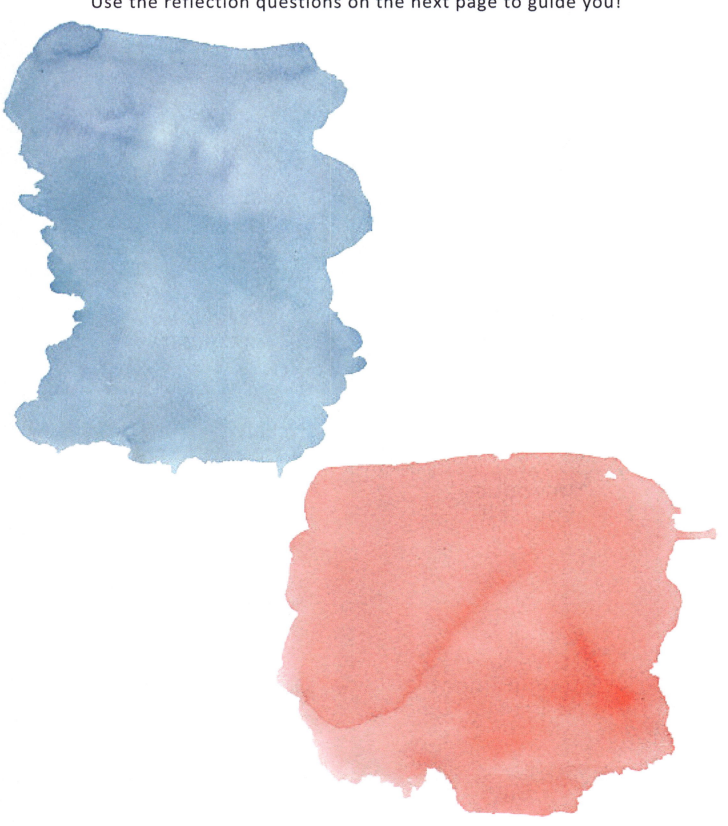

Laminate and cut out the following communication skills cards. Chose 1-2 to practice with a loved one. Remember, learning communication skills takes practice, but you can do it!

Make eye contact	Ask a question
Say no (assertively)	Make a request
Introduce yourself	Initiate a conversation
Give a compliment	Receive a compliment

Communication skills cards cont.

Say "I'm sorry"	Use an "I" statement
Voice your opinion (assertively)	Admit you made a mistake
Ask for help	Set a boundary with someone
Make a phone call	Ask an employee a question (at a store, restaurant)

Reflection

What did you learn about social skills and communicating with others? How did this lesson add to the knowledge you already had? What questions do you still have? Can you describe the different types of communication and give examples from your own life? Name one thing you can do to begin improving your ability to communicate well with others. How will this improve your relationships with others? How will this honor God? Which social skills exercise was the most impactful?

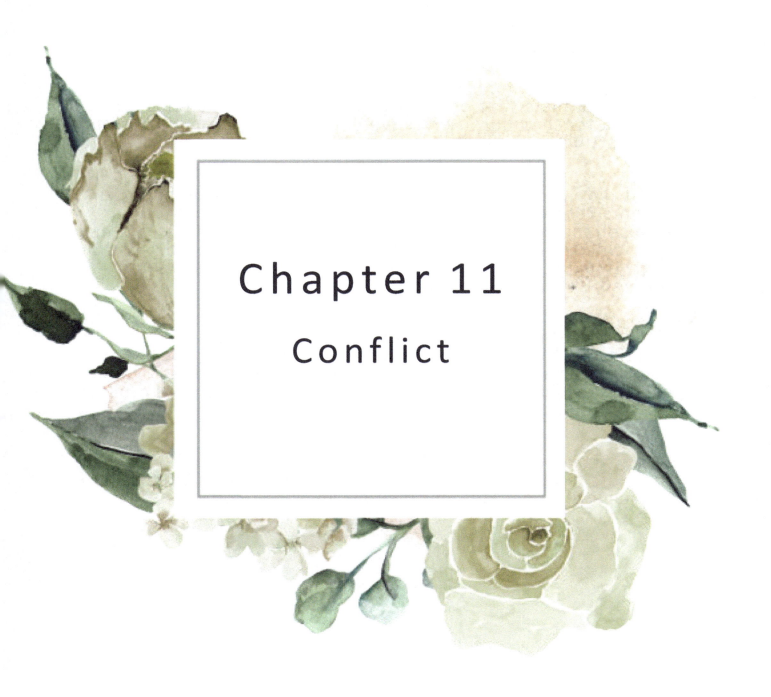

Chapter 11
Conflict

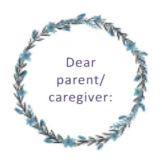

Dear parent/caregiver:

A conflict can occur when we do not agree with someone else. Conflict is inevitable, but how we manage conflict in our home will impact our children long-term. This lesson will explore typical conflicts that occur between children. It is important to actively teach children effective conflict resolution skills rather than letting them figure it out on their own.

What did you learn about conflict growing up? How did your parents resolve conflict in the home? How do you and your spouse resolve conflict? How do you manage conflict between your children? We often model ways to mange conflict without even thinking about it. Conflict resolution skills as well as problem-solving skills will be explored in this curriculum.

If there are high levels of conflict in your home, I suggest meeting with a therapist. Sometimes specific tools designed for your unique situation are needed. This book addresses general conflict resolution skills, but problems of a more severe nature warrant additional help.

Parent/caregiver journal: Take some time to journal your thoughts about how you manage conflict. What factors in your life have played a role in how you approach conflict? Take some time to explore these feelings and share with a therapist or a loved one.

A conflict can occur when we disagree with someone else. There are many helpful ways we can resolve conflict, but many unhelpful ways too. What are some unhelpful ways?

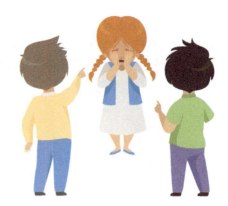

How can I resolve conflict with others?

Instead of blaming, and saying things like "You made me angry," you can use "I" statements.

I felt _____ when _____ happened.

What I need from you is

_____

_____

Sometimes we need to state our needs when we are communicating with others.

Am I taking responsibility for my role in the conflict? Am I addressing the other person's feelings? Am I listening to their side of the story too?

"Pleasant words are like a honeycomb. They make a person happy and healthy." Proverbs 16:24 (ICB)

You are playing with a friend and he takes your toy. You quickly became angry and your first thought is to take it back or hit him. Write or draw two healthy ways you can manage your anger. (Ask a trusted adult for help if needed!)

You are playing with a group of friends and one child starts teasing another one. What should you do? Remember what we learned about how we should treat each other? Look at the following picture. How do you think the little boy feels? Is this behavior honoring God?

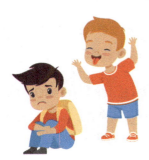

As you are learning how to manage conflict with others, remember it is important to ask an adult for help if you need.

One of the first steps I can take when a conflict occurs is identifying my feelings about it. Think back to everything we've learned so far about our emotions. What emotions are you experiencing during conflict and where do you feel them in your body? Write down your thoughts here.

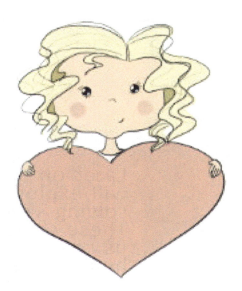

Sometimes, one of the most helpful ways to resolve conflict is showing empathy for the other person. It is easy to become consumed with our thoughts, feelings, and needs. Empathy is when we are able to consider how another person is feeling. How can having empathy for another person help us resolve conflict?

Another thing to consider is where the conflict is coming from. Are my feelings based on fact or am I making assumptions about the situation? Do I need to ask questions to clarify something? What else do I need to understand the situation completely before I react? Am I being assertive in my communication or aggressive? Am I more worried about winning an argument or maintaining my friendship?

How can the anger management and communication skills we learned earlier help us resolve conflict with others?

_____

_____

_____

Later on in this book, we will explore problem-solving skills in depth. These skills can also help us resolve conflict in a healthy manner.

Write down a time you had conflict with someone else. What happened? What did you say and do? What did the other person say and do? Is there something you can improve? What was helpful and unhelpful? Be specific in identifying your thoughts, feelings, and reactions during the conflict. Remember, we can look at past experiences, learn from them, and see them as opportunities to grow.

_____

_____

_____

_____

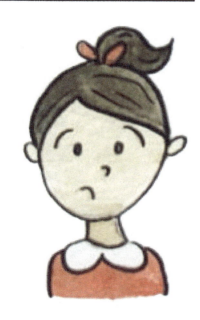

"Don't ever stop being kind and truthful. Let kindness and truth show in all you do. Write them down in your mind as if on a tablet. Then you will be respected and pleasing to both God and men."

Proverbs 3:3-4 (ICB)

Think back to the list of emotions at the beginning of this book. Which emotions make a conflict worse? Which ones are more helpful? How about the communication skills we learned? Which skills help the situation? Which ones make it worse? How can I calm down before reacting to a stressful situation? Draw or write your thoughts here.

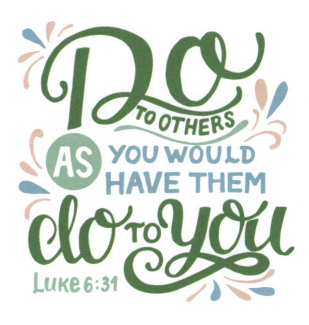

Sometimes a helpful tool to learn a new skill is a role play. Choose an issue you're working on resolving and ask a trusted adult or friend to help you act it out. This is a great way to practice what you want to say and how you want to say it. It's okay if you make mistakes, this is the best time to practice! You can also act out the issue using puppets and practice what you'd like to say.

After your initial role play, try it again, but from the other person's point of view. How can seeing it from their perspective help you understand them better?

Draw a picture of what you learned during your role play.

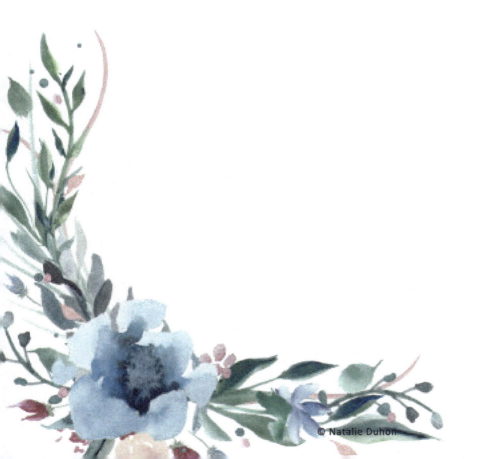

Take some time to write or draw your thoughts about this chapter.
Use the reflection questions on the next page to guide you!

Reflection

What did you learn about conflict? How did this lesson add to the knowledge you already had about managing conflict with others? What questions do you still have? Name one step you can take when a conflict with someone else occurs. How can managing conflict appropriately honor God and others?

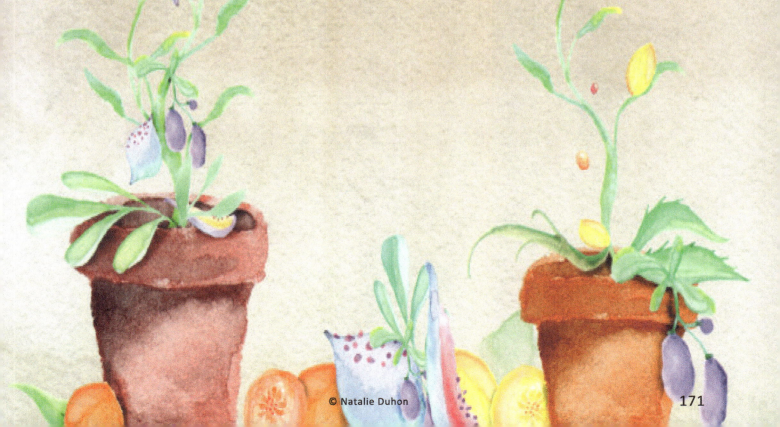

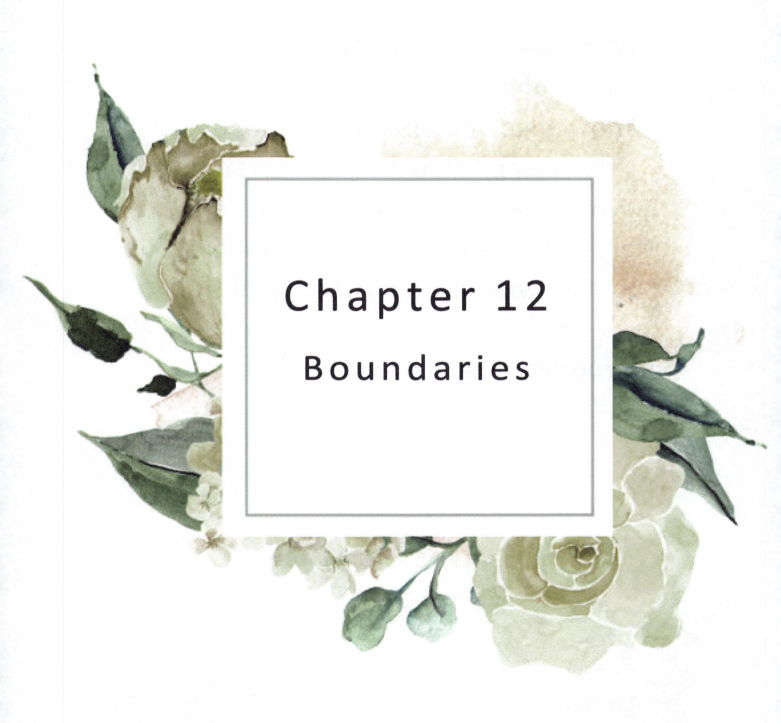

Chapter 12
Boundaries

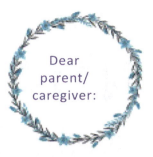

Dear parent/caregiver:

Teaching young children boundaries is an important aspect of their safety and the safety of others. Every family has their own idea about personal space. This is an important concept to teach and model for your child. Boundaries include more than just physical boundaries. They also include emotional boundaries and being able to assert oneself in difficult situations. It is important that we model appropriate emotional and physical boundaries to our children. We can help them by respecting their boundaries and teaching them to respect the boundaries of themselves and others.

One way we can teach our children good boundaries is asking them before we hug them. This helps them learn that their body belongs to them and they have the right to say no. We can also let well-meaning family members know if our child does not like to be hugged. Advocating for our child at a young age can go a long way in his/her emotional development. There are many great resources that teach proper human anatomy and consent. This will also help them learn how they can stay safe and how to recognize an unsafe situation. (Be sure your child has your phone number memorized).

It is helpful to pick a couple of trustworthy people in your child's life that he/she can talk to if ever in an unsafe situation. The topic of boundaries has often been neglected in the past, but it is important to have this talk with your child regularly. These talks need to begin at a young age and continue well into your child's teenage years.

Parent/caregiver Journal: What were you taught about boundaries? Were you taught that you have to hug others? Were you taught that you can't say no or be rude? Do you feel like you are able to set healthy boundaries with others as an adult? Share these thoughts with a loved one, a pastor, or a therapist.

BOUNDARIES

Personal space between two people is important. Just like a fence separates two pieces of land, I need to set an invisible boundary between myself and others. If I ever feel unsafe or uncomfortable, I can let a trusted adult know! Who are the trusted adults in my life? My body is mine only and I have the right to set boundaries with others. My body belongs to ME.

I can say no to hugs. I can wave, smile, or shake hands. I don't have to hug someone else, but I can still be respectful and polite. When setting boundaries, I need to be direct and firm. If I ever feel unsafe or uncomfortable, I will tell a trusted adult right away.

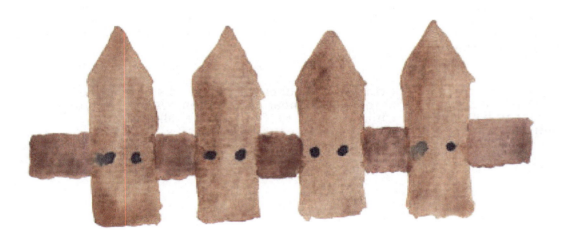

Write down a list of your trusted adults here. (It is also helpful to have their phone numbers memorized).

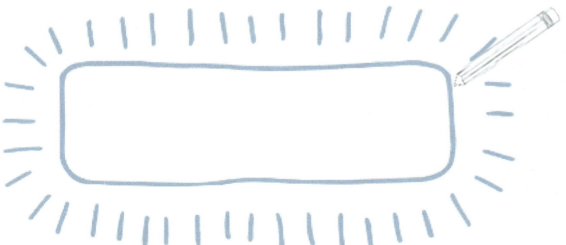

Let's go back to our emotion words for a moment. Some words to describe how we feel when we need to set a boundary with someone include uneasy, nervous, or apprehensive. Remember to listen to your body and what it's trying to tell you. God gave us instincts and emotions for a reason. We can learn how to listen to our body with practice.

These uncomfortable feelings tell us that something is not right and we need to ask for help. What words can you use to describe when you're feeling uncomfortable?

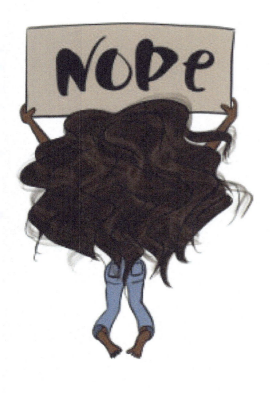

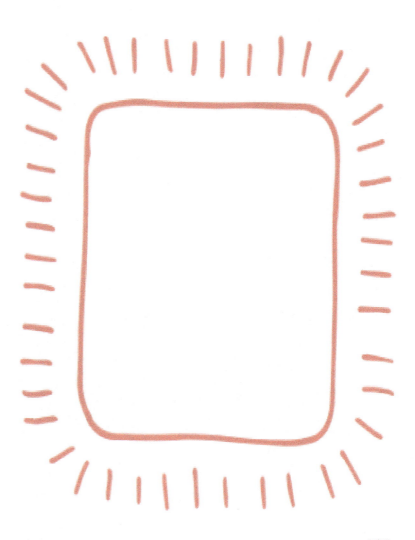

I also need to respect the boundaries of others. This includes respecting their body and their belongings. If they do not want to hug me, they do not have to. If someone tells me to stop doing something, I need to be respectful and listen. I also need to remember that I cannot touch or take something that does not belong to me. That is called stealing and it is not okay. Write down some ways you can be respectful of another person's boundaries.

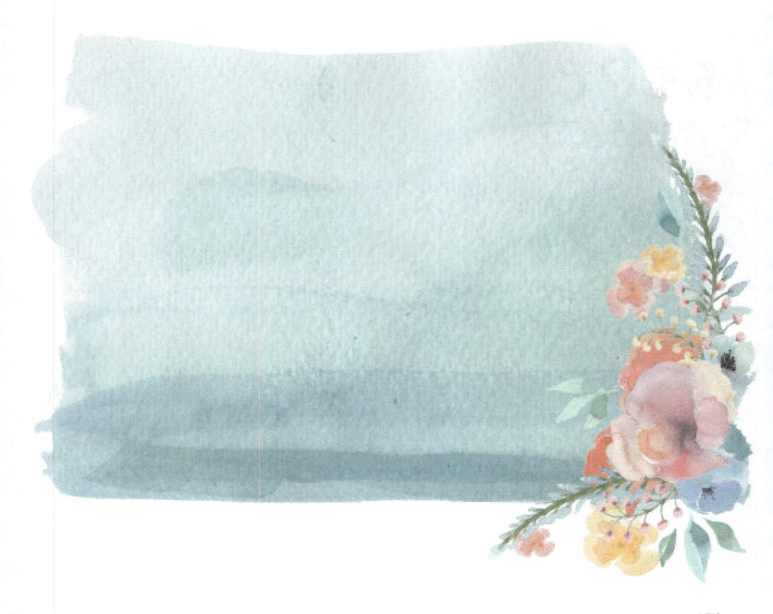

Did you know that boundaries don't just include physical boundaries? Having good boundaries also includes emotional boundaries!

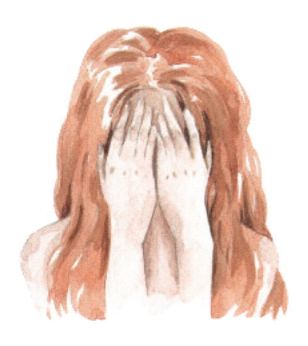

If someone tells us they need some time alone or they ask us to respect their feelings, it is important to do so. We also need to set boundaries with others when we need some space. If we need to take a minute to calm down and think, it is okay to tell another person that we need a break.

We can tell someone if they hurt our feelings. If we hurt their feelings, we can be respectful and listen when they tell us about it.

Remember when we learned about communication styles? It is important to be assertive when setting boundaries with others. We don't want to be afraid to say no when it comes to protecting our bodies and our emotions. Being polite does not mean letting people take advantage of us. Now is a good time to do a role play and practice setting boundaries with others. Write down what you learned here. Examples can include: saying no to a hug, asking for space (physical or emotional), etc.

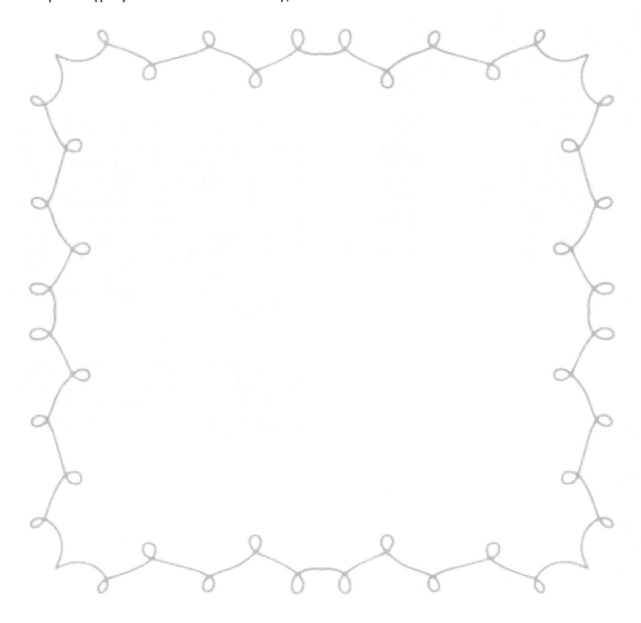

Let's explore some examples of healthy and unhealthy boundaries. Circle the correct answer.

1. My friend and I are wrestling and having fun. Suddenly she tells me to stop. I think she's playing so I keep wrestling. Am I being respectful of the boundary she has set? How can I respect her decision?

2. I see an old friend and try to hug her. She says she doesn't want to hug right now. I respect her decision and politely say hi instead. Am I being respectful of her boundaries?

3. My new friend shows me his new backpack and all of his cool toys. Without asking, I open the backpack to see what's inside. Is this being respectful of my friend's property?

4. I hurt my friend's feelings and I'm trying to apologize to him. He tells me he's upset and needs some space. Instead of being respectful of his need for some space, I keep telling him I'm sorry and he needs to forgive me. How can I be more respectful of his boundaries?

5. I see my friend's journal on her desk when I go to her house. Would reading it be a violation of her boundaries? Discuss why.

© Natalie Duhon

Take some time to write or draw your thoughts about this chapter.
Use the reflection questions on the next page to guide you!

Reflection

What did you learn about boundaries?
How did this lesson add to the knowledge you already had about boundaries?
What questions do you still have?
Where do you need to set healthy boundaries?
How do you react when another person sets boundaries with you?
What is the importance of setting boundaries with others?

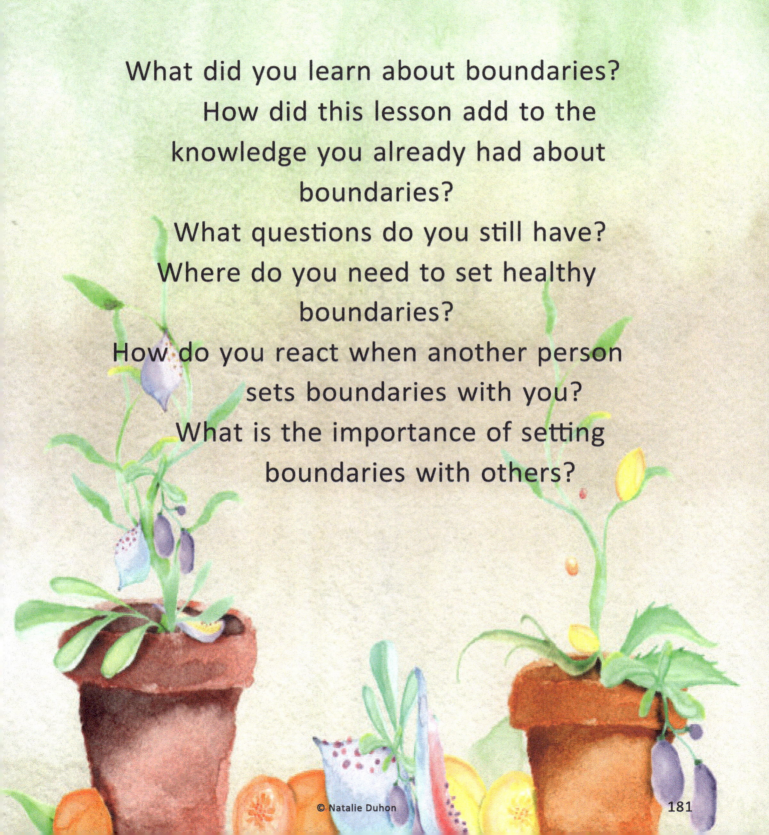

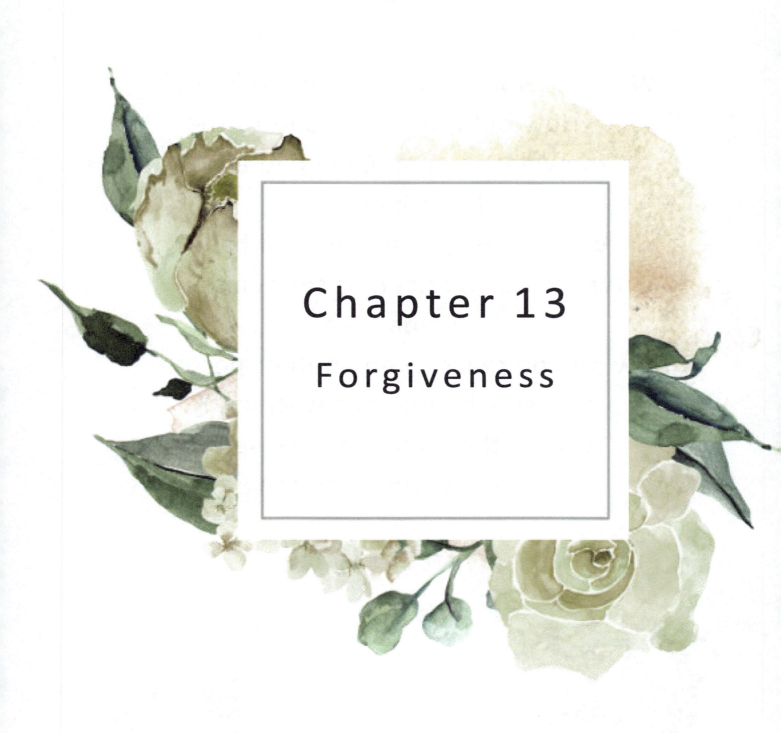
Chapter 13
Forgiveness

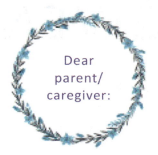

Dear parent/caregiver:

The chapter on forgiveness in this book will focus on issues such as a child taking away a toy or hurting a friend's feelings. This is NOT a resource designed to discuss forgiving issues of a more severe nature. These should be processed with a pastor or licensed therapist. Children should be taught about forgiveness, but they should also learn appropriate boundary setting. Enduring any form of abuse or neglect is not okay.

FORGIVENESS

I can learn to forgive if I ask Jesus to help me. Forgiving someone means I accept their apology. It doesn't mean I allow them to hurt me. Let's turn to the Bible to learn about God's definition of forgiveness. Copy the following Bible verse.

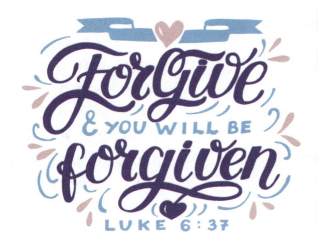

_____

_____

_____

_____

In Mark 11:25-26 (ICB), **Jesus tells us:"When you are praying, and you remember that you are angry with another person about something, then forgive him. If you do this, then your Father in heaven will also forgive your sins. But if you don't forgive other people, then your Father in heaven will not forgive your sins."**

"Do not be angry with each other, but forgive each other. If someone does wrong to you, then forgive him. Forgive each other because the Lord forgave you. Do all these things; but most important, love each other. Love is what holds you all together in perfect unity. Let the peace that Christ gives control your thinking. You were all called together in one body to have peace. Always be thankful." Colossians 3:13-15

What does forgiveness mean to you? What does unity look like? What about peace? Discuss these traits with a loved one.

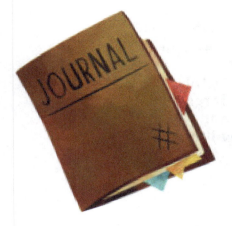

Is there someone you need to ask to forgive you? Is there someone you need to forgive? (Remember, forgiving someone doesn't mean you continue allowing them to treat you poorly. Forgiveness is between you and God). Journal your thoughts here and pray about how you can work on asking for forgiveness or how you can forgive someone else.

_____

_____

_____

_____

"Jesus answered, "I tell you, you must forgive him more than 7 times. You must forgive him even if he does wrong to you 70 times 7." Matthew 18:22 (ICB)

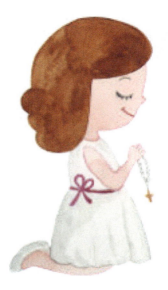

Dear God,

Please help me forgive other people when they hurt my feelings. Remind me that just as you forgave me, I should also forgive them. Please help me learn from my mistakes and treat other people the way I want to be treated. Please help me be quick to forgive when I hurt others.

Write your own prayer here. Or choose a Bible verse about forgiveness that you can copy and memorize.

_____

_____

_____

_____

Remember, forgiveness does NOT mean letting other people treat us poorly. We need to set healthy boundaries with them, but we can still offer forgiveness. Ask a trusted adult if you need help with this and ALWAYS tell them if you or someone you know is being mistreated.

Take some time to write or draw your thoughts about this chapter.
Use the reflection questions on the next page to guide you!

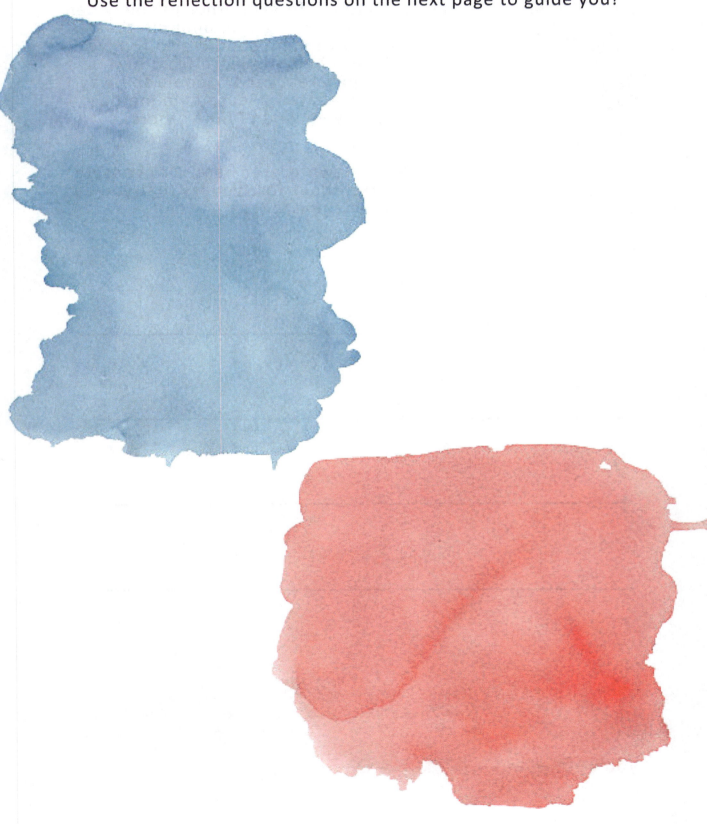

Reflection

What did you learn about forgiveness? How did this lesson add to the knowledge you already had about forgiveness? What questions do you still have? Is there someone you need to forgive? Do you need to ask anyone for forgiveness? Why is it important to apologize when you are wrong? Look up the definition of forgiveness, then find out what the Bible says. What are the similarities and differences?

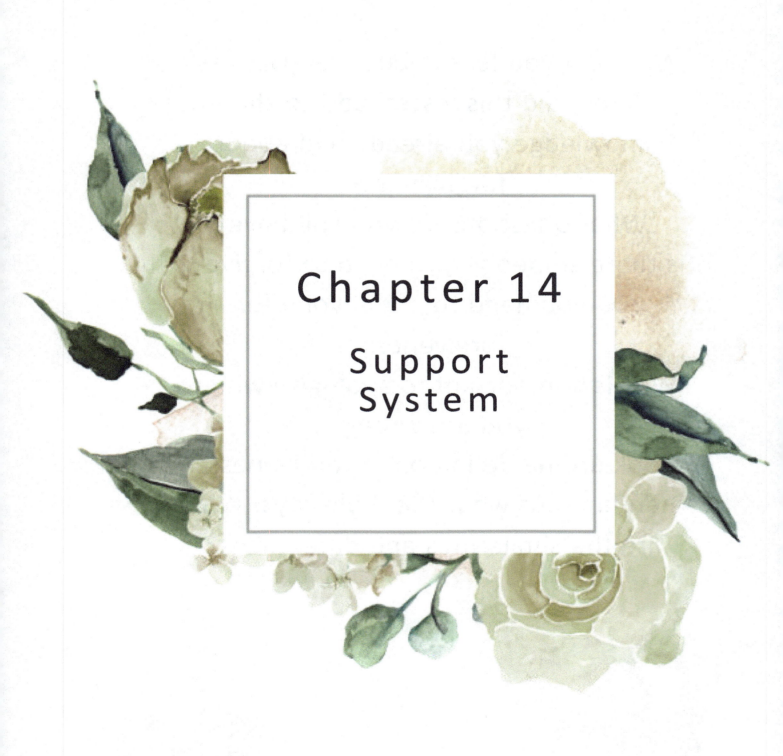

Chapter 14

Support System

SUPPORT SYSTEM

God created us for fellowship, not to live life alone. At the beginning of creation, God didn't want Adam to be alone, so He created Eve. Who helps inspire me to grow closer to God?

- neighbors
- family
- friends
- parents/caregivers
- church leaders
- homeschool groups

"An enemy might defeat one person, but two people together can defend themselves. A rope that has three parts wrapped together is hard to break." Ecclesiastes 4:12 (ICB)

Draw and write down the names of specific people in your life who love and support you. Have you told them how much you appreciate them? After you draw them, say a prayer for your loved ones. You can also create a thank you card for them!

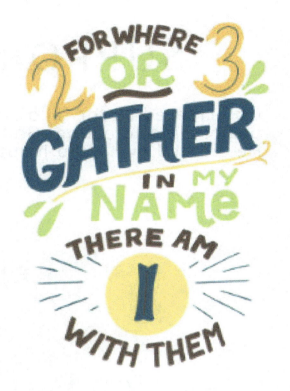

"Two people are better than one. They get more done by working together. If one person falls, the other can help him up. But it is bad for the person who is alone when he falls. No one is there to help him." Ecclesiastes 4:9-10 (ICB)

"Iron can sharpen iron. In the same way, people can help each other." Proverbs 27:17 (ICB)

Pick five people whom you look up to and ask them their favorite Bible verse. Ask them to share why that verse holds significance for them. Choose one or two to write here:

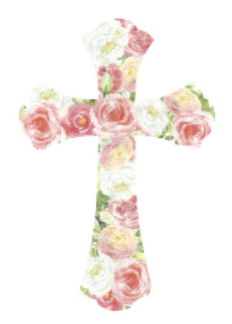

_____

_____

_____

_____

What are some qualities that make a person a good friend? How can I be a good friend? Write down your thoughts here. What does the Bible teach us?

"Some friends may ruin you. But a real friend will be more loyal than a brother." Proverbs 18:24

"Whenever you are able, do good to people who need help." Proverbs 3:27 (ICB)

"An evil person causes trouble. And a person who gossips ruins friendships." Proverbs 16:28 (ICB)

"Whoever spends time with wise people will become wise. But whoever makes friends with fools will suffer." Proverbs 13:20 (ICB)

Take some time to write or draw your thoughts about this chapter. Use the reflection questions on the next page to guide you!

Reflection

Why is it important to have a healthy support system?

Who are the members of your support system? How do they help you?

How did this lesson add to the knowledge you already had?

What questions do you still have?

What does the Bible say about our relationships with others and leaning on each other for support?

Is there someone in your life who needs your support? How can you help them?

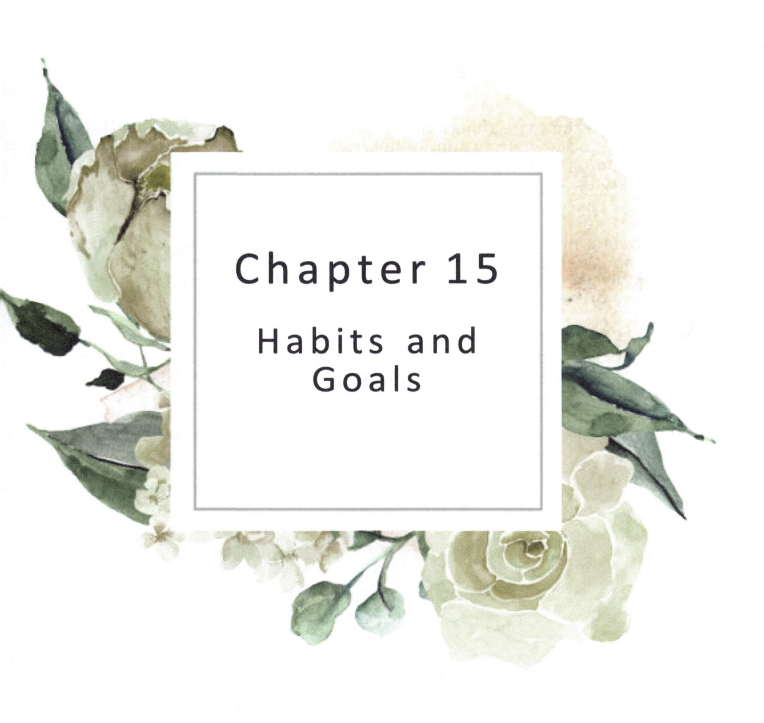

Chapter 15

Habits and Goals

How Do Habits and Goals Shape Our Life?

Habits are the little things we do on a regular basis, usually without thinking about it. They can be helpful or unhelpful, depending on the habit! An unhelpful habit would be biting our fingernails. A helpful habit would be automatically saying "please" and "thank you."

Our habits impact our goals in life. A goal is something we want to accomplish. These can be short-term goals (to be completed in a week or a month) and long-term goals (to be completed in a few months or even years!)

A short-term goal might be to complete five lessons in your math book. A long-term goal is for you to finish your current grade!

It is helpful to understand how our goals line up with the Word of God.

> "A person may think up plans. But the Lord decides what he will do." Proverbs 16:9 (ICB)

What direction do my choices and actions lead to? Are my goals in line with God's plan for my life? Am I trying to please God or others? What does the Bible say?

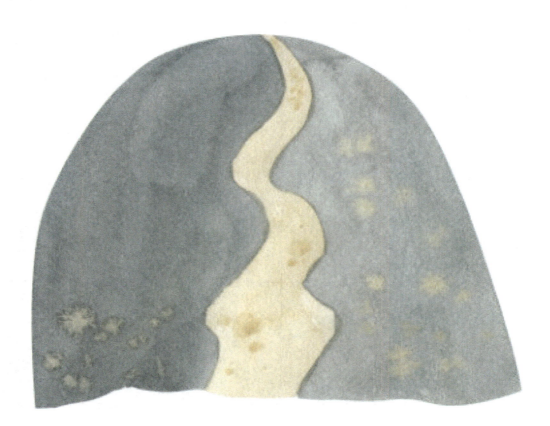

"Enter through the narrow gate. The road that leads to hell is a very easy road. And the gate to hell is very wide. Many people enter through that gate. But the gate that opens the way to true life is very small. And the road to true life is very hard. Only a few people find that road." Matthew 7:13-14 (ICB)

Daily Habits Tracker

	Sunday	Monday	Tuesday	Wednesday	Thursday	Friday	Saturday
Pray							
Read Bible							
Brush teeth							
Bath/shower							
Exercise							
Eat healthy							
Finish schoolwork							
Chores							
Thank God							

How do I set goals and why are they important? Who/what can help me achieve them? Am I letting God have a say in my goals or do I try to do things my own way? Am I letting the world be my guide or God?

Complete the goal sheet on the next page. How are my daily activities helping me work toward my short-term and long-term goals? How are these activities helping or hurting my mental health? What do I need to add to my daily activities?

"Trust the Lord with all your heart. Don't depend on your own understanding." Proverbs 3:5 (ICB)

Write down your goal for each day. Pray for each one and ask God for you to accomplish His will.

Sunday _____

Monday _____

Tuesday _____

Wednesday _____

Thursday _____

Friday _____

Saturday _____

"Guide my steps as you promised. Don't let any sin control me." Psalm 119:133 (ICB)

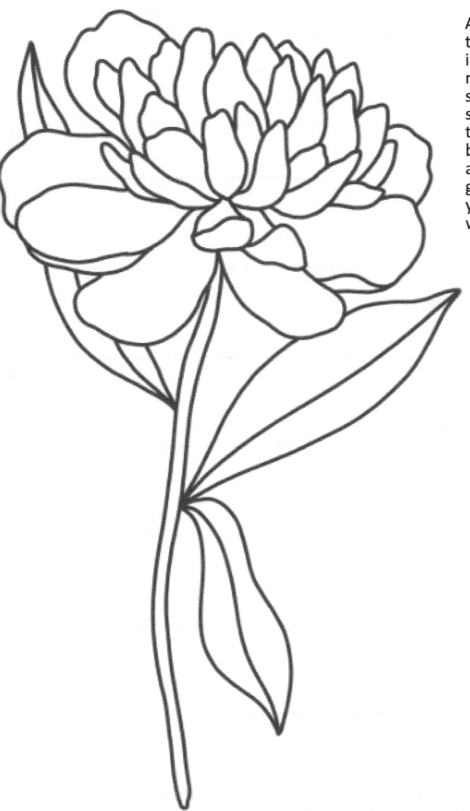

A plant needs several things to grow. These include air, water, nutrients, and sunshine. What are some things you need to grow? (These can be physical, spiritual, and emotional growth). Write down your ideas and share with a loved one.

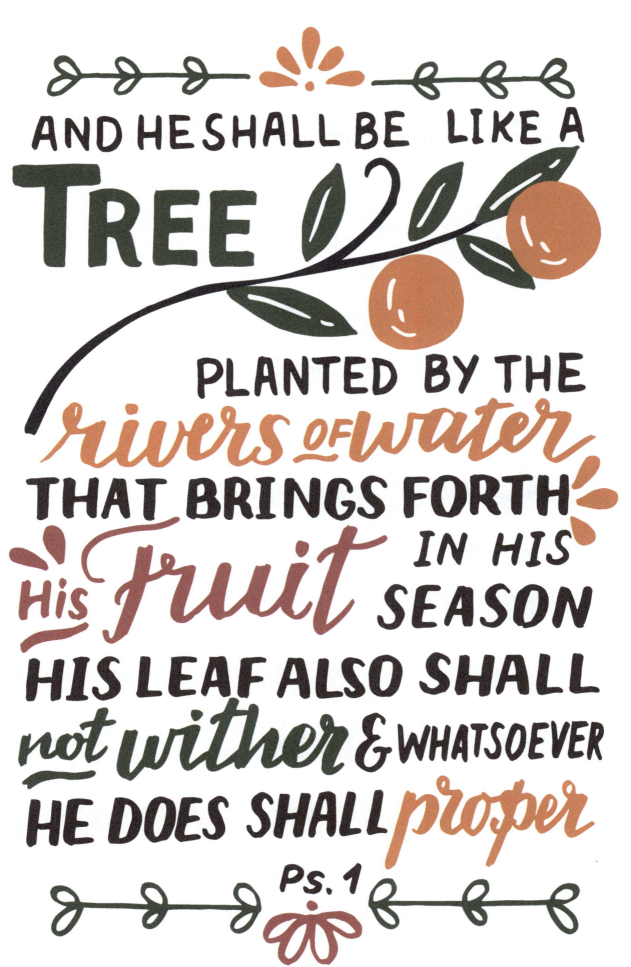

Take some time to write or draw your thoughts about this chapter.
Use the reflection questions on the next page to guide you!

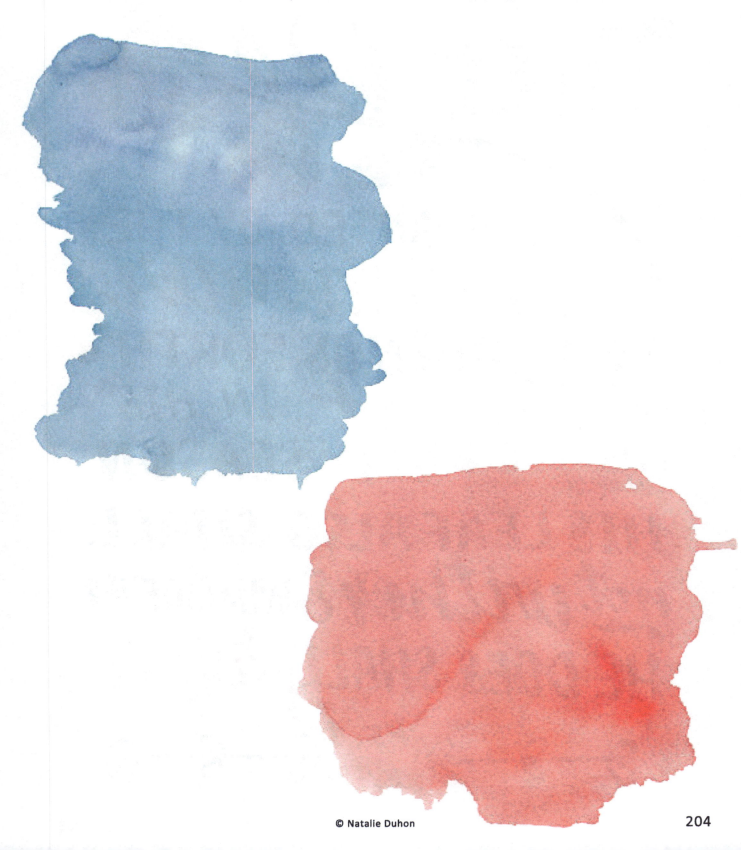

Reflection

What did you learn about habits/goals?
How did this lesson add to the knowledge you already had?
What questions do you still have?
What's one habit you want to change?
What's one goal you want to start working on?
What is the first step you need to take?

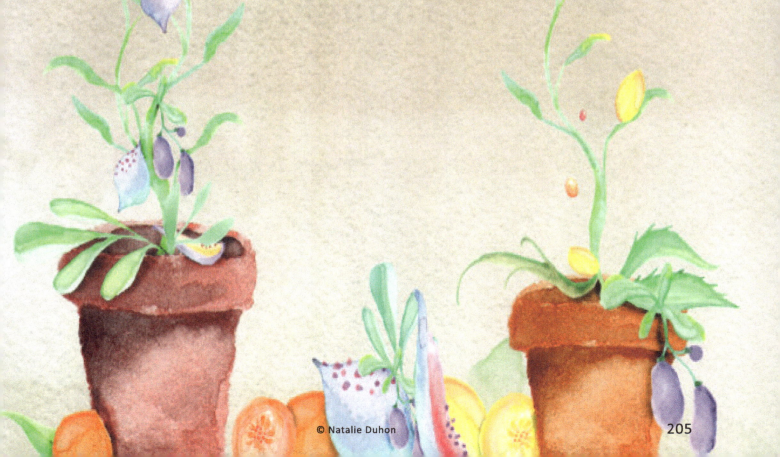

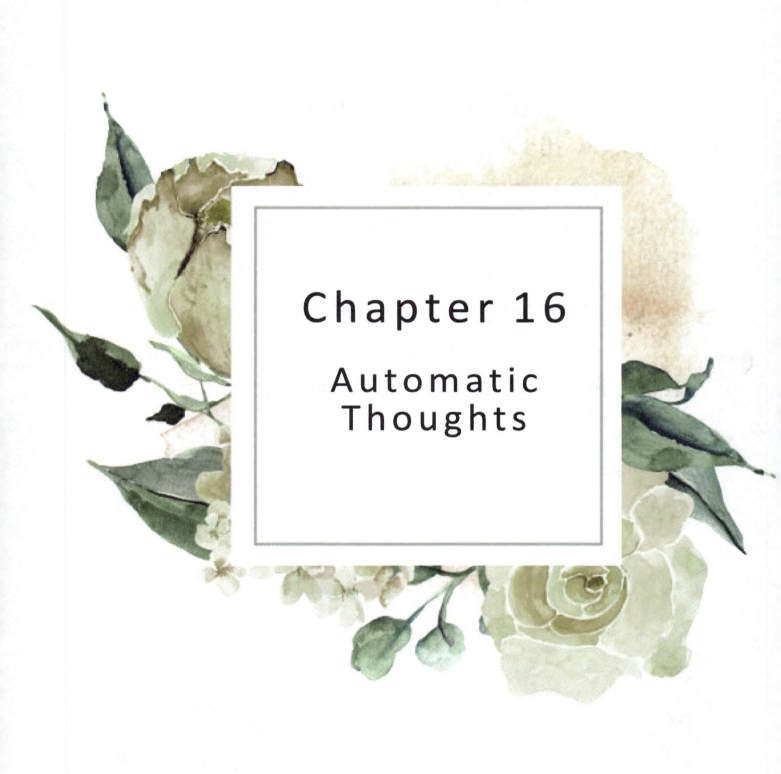

Chapter 16

Automatic Thoughts

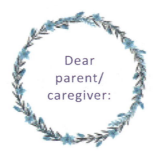

Dear parent/caregiver:

Throughout our lives, we constantly receive messages from the people in our environment. These can include family, friends, teachers, and others in our community. It can also include what we read in books, magazines, and see on television. Social media also plays a role in our thought process.

What messages did you hearing growing up? What messages have become your "automatic thoughts?" Are they positive or negative? Examples may include: "I'm not good enough," "I'm not pretty enough," "I'll never succeed," or "I'm not smart enough." When we have these thoughts regularly, we are more likely to experience sadness, worry, or anger. These messages can have a lasting impact on our mental health.

We can also have positive or more realistic thoughts. We don't want to discount negative experiences, but we do want to be realistic and balanced in our thinking. Examples include "This will be hard, but I can do this," "I am a worthy person who is loved by God," and "I've faced a similar problem before and I have the skills to cope now."

If you struggle with negative thoughts, seeing a therapist of your own would be extremely beneficial. It can also help you understand how what we say and do as parents/caregivers can greatly impact the thought processes of our children.

*This is not to make parents/caregivers feel guilty. We are not perfect and will make mistakes. When our children see us growing and acknowledging our mistakes, they will feel more comfortable asking for help when they need. When they see our need for God's grace, they will better understand their need for God's grace.

Bible memorization can help us and our children focus our thoughts on what is truly important.

Parent/caregiver journal: Take time to journal some of these negative thoughts that you've experienced. Discuss with a loved one, a pastor, or a therapist.

© Natalie Duhon

Automatic Thoughts

We can have so many thoughts in our mind, that we sometimes lose track! We experience thoughts without even thinking about them. One way to describe them is automatic thoughts. It's important to be aware of these thoughts and determine whether they are in line with God's word or the world. Writing them down can help us recognize any patterns in our thinking. (Fear of failure is one).

"We capture every thought and make it give up and obey Christ." 2 Cor 10:5 ICB

Our thoughts have a major impact on our feelings. However, we know that our feelings do not always give us an accurate picture of our situation. Sometimes our thoughts may be negative, which may cause us to feel unhappy. Examples would be thinking "I'm not good enough," "I'm not smart enough," or "I never do anything right." If we've been reading our Bible, we know that these are NOT true!

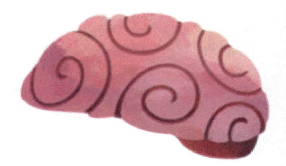

Situation: I walk into a room where my friends are playing, say hi, and no one acknowledges me.

Thought 1: No one likes me. → I feel sad, hurt, and my self-esteem decreases.

Thought 2: They're rude. → I feel angry, frustrated, and resentful.

Thought 3: They're busy and didn't hear me. → I don't have any strong feelings about it.

The situation is the exact same, but my thoughts have a direct impact on my feelings. My feelings can have a major impact on my behavior, so it's important that I am aware of my thoughts!

"Be very careful about what you think. Your thoughts run your life."
Proverbs 4:23 (ICB)

> "Do not be shaped by this world. Instead be changed within by a new way of thinking. Then you will be able to decide what God wants for you. And you will be able to know what is good and pleasing to God and what is perfect."
> Romans 12:2 (ICB)

Situation: My good friend is ignoring me.

Thought 1: She doesn't want to be my friend anymore. → Sad

Thought 2: She is mean and rude. → Angry

Thought 3: Maybe she is upset. → Compassion

Thought 4: Maybe she's sick. → Concern, worry

Thought 5: Maybe she didn't hear me. → No change in feelings; neutral

> "Brothers, continue to think about the things that are good and worthy of praise. Think about the things that are true and honorable and right and pure and beautiful and respected."
> Phil 4:8 (ICB)

Over the next week, pay attention to how your thoughts relate to your feelings. Pay attention to what you are thinking and feeling at different parts of the day, during different circumstances. Write them down here. Remember, this will take practice! Always check your thoughts against the word of God, our ultimate authority!

Situation	Thought	Feeling

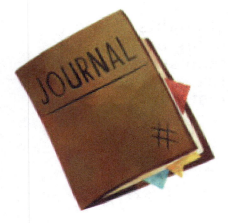

What's your favorite subject? How does it connect to God? How does it bring you joy? What does it teach you about God? Journal your thoughts here.

_____

_____

_____

_____

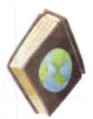
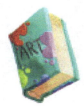

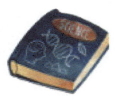
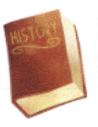

Have you ever felt like things were out of your control? Maybe your day started off wrong and continued to get worse.

Think about the differences between things in your life that you have control over and things that you do not. Write them here.

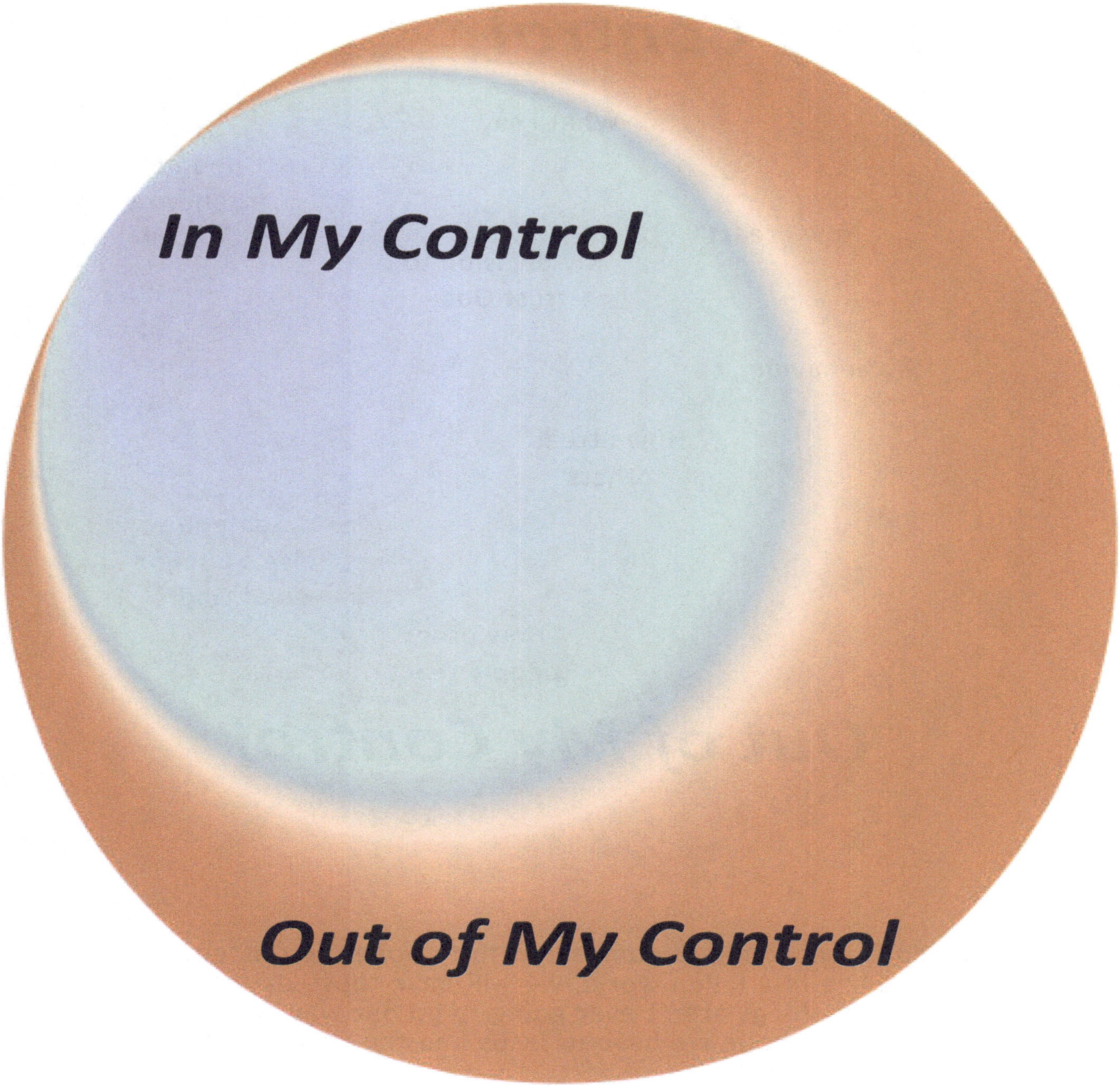

In My Control

Out of My Control

Hymn: My Hope Is Built On Nothing Less (On Christ The Solid Rock I Stand)

In My Control

- My thoughts
- What I say
- How I react
- My decision to trust God
- My behavior
- How I treat others

Out of My Control

- Other people's thoughts
- Other people's behavior
- What other people say/do
- Someone else's opinion of God
- How other people react

How do these examples compare with the ones you listed? Since we live in a fallen world, we will have those days where we feel that things aren't ever going to go our way. We can hold on to the hope we have in Jesus and the promise of eternity in Heaven.

© Natalie Duhon

Take some time to write or draw your thoughts about this chapter.
Use the reflection questions on the next page to guide you!

Reflection

What did you learn about automatic thoughts?

How did this lesson add to the knowledge you already had?

What questions do you still have?

Name one thing you can do to begin identifying your automatic thoughts. How can this help you?

There are many verses in the Bible that teach us about how to manage our thoughts. Which one stands out to you the most?

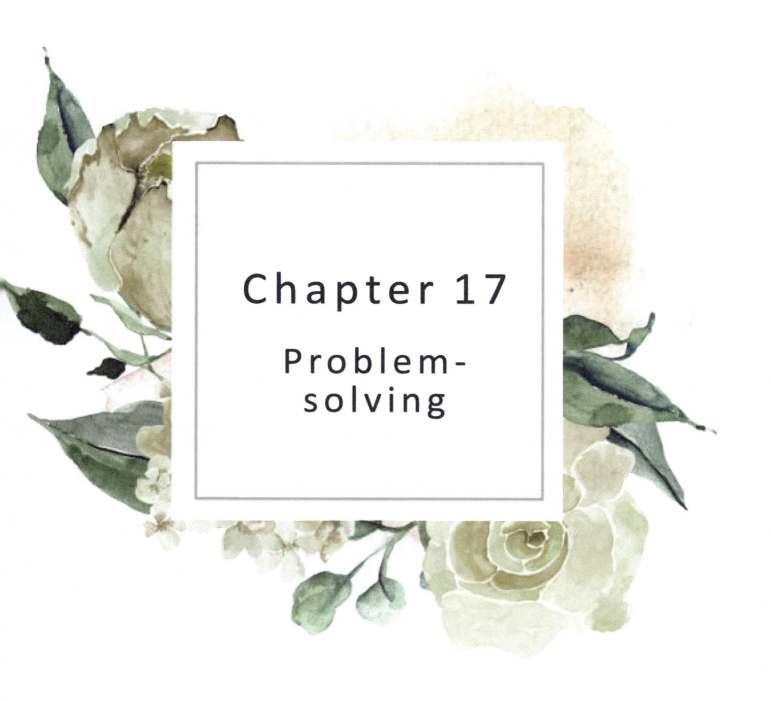

Chapter 17
Problem-solving

Problem-Solving

Step 1-Identify the problem.

Step 2-What can I do on my own? What do I need help with?

Step 3-What result am I hoping for?

Step 4-Explore different ways to solve the problem.

Step 5-Pick one and try it!

Step 1-Identify the problem (be as specific as possible).

It is important to list details about your current problem. Who/what is involved? What's in my control? What's out of my control? Am I focusing on something that's a current problem or is it something from the past that's unresolved? What thoughts and feelings do I have about this problem? Am I focusing on one problem or multiple problems? (It is helpful to focus on one thing at a time).

Step 2-What can I do on my own? What do I need help with?

Who can I ask to help me with this problem? (Don't forget to pray and ask God for help). Have I encountered a similar problem in the past? What was helpful/unhelpful then? Have I gained new knowledge or skills since that time?

Step 3-What result am I hoping for?

Is it in line with God's word? How will my decisions impact others? How will solving this problem help me? What impact will this problem have if it remains unsolved?

Step 4-Explore different ways to solve the problem.

What do I think will be the most helpful? (Try to think of several different ways to solve the problem. Then evaluate which one makes the most sense). List possible steps for the ones that seem most helpful. Are they doable?

Step 5-Pick one and try it! Did it help? What could I have done differently? Remember, each problem we encounter is a learning opportunity!

> Use the next two pages to identify a current problem and try practicing these problem-solving steps. Or, you can think about how you solved a past problem. Remember, it takes practice!

© Natalie Duhon

Problem-Solving

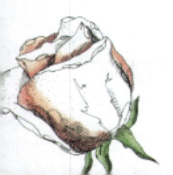

Problem-Solving

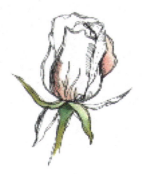

Take some time to write or draw your thoughts about this chapter.
Use the reflection questions on the next page to guide you!

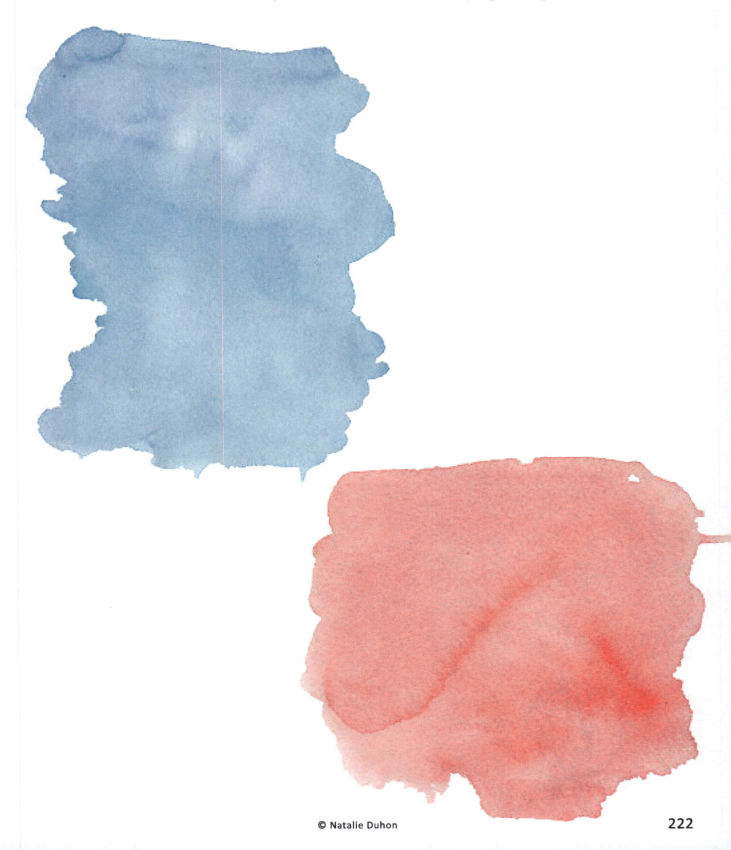

Reflection

What did you learn about problem-solving?
How did this lesson add to the knowledge you already had?
What questions do you still have?
How have you solved problems in the past? What can you do differently this time?
When faced with a problem, does prayer tend to be first or last on your problem-solving list?

Chapter 18
Coping Skills

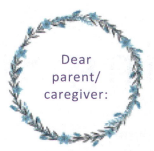

Dear parent/caregiver:

We all learn various ways to cope with stress, whether or not we are taught them. Unfortunately, if we are not taught healthy coping skills, we may fall into the trap of using unhealthy coping skills. Some of these may be nervous habits like biting our nails or fidgeting. Other unhealthy coping skills can be detrimental to our health.

Examples include: drug or alcohol abuse, excessive spending or gambling, isolation, ruminating thoughts, comparing ourselves to others, etc.

Relationships can also be impacted when we engage in behaviors such as blaming, silent treatment, and denial. Sometimes our habits don't cause us much trouble, but they can severely impact our functioning if we let them get out of control. If your child's behavior is impacting their functioning, it is highly advised that they see a therapist. (These can include, but are not limited to, changes in behavior, hygiene, grades, and relationships with others).

Coping Skills

Coping skills are healthy activities we can do that help us feel better when we're upset. Always ask yourself if they're honoring God. Let's use the alphabet to brainstorm lots of ways to feel better! On a separate sheet of paper, write or draw a way to improve your mood for each letter. (Example: for the letter "A," we can work on an art project).

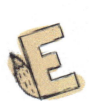
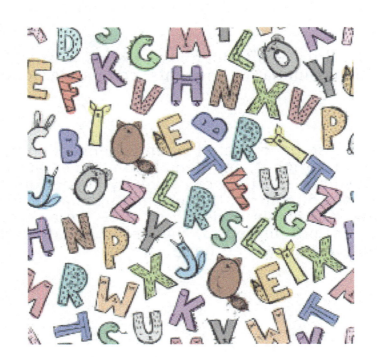
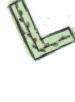

Here are some examples: Listen to an audio book, create something using chalk, clean up your environment, try a new hobby, do some stretches, go to the library.

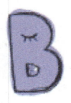
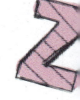

Which one is most helpful to you? Which one would you like to try? What do you need to try it? Ask a loved one for help if needed. (Example: if art is helpful, you may want to ask a loved one to help you buy supplies.)

© Natalie Duhon

Cut out and laminate. Act out each coping skill and have a friend guess. You can use these or draw your own. (Or print two copies of each page and play memory)

Swimming	Talk to someone
Listen to music	Time with a pet
Read	Dance
Sing	Walk

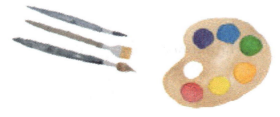

Intentionally left blank for double sided printing

Cut out and laminate. Act out each coping skill and have a friend guess. You can use these or draw your own. (Or print two copies of each page and play memory)

Ride a bike	Sit outside
Draw a picture	Journal
Take a shower or bath	Pray
Read the Bible	Church

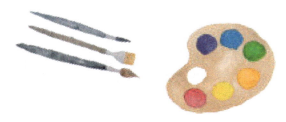

Intentionally left blank for double sided printing

Cut out and laminate. Act out each coping skill and have a friend guess. You can use these or draw your own. (Or print two copies of each page and play memory)

Call someone	Deep breathing
Swing	Make up your own
Gardening	Play a game
Sports	Set boundaries

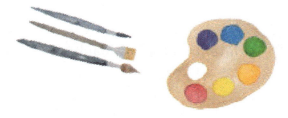

Intentionally left blank for double sided printing

Cut out and laminate. Act out each coping skill and have a friend guess. You can use these or draw your own. (Or print two copies of each page and play memory)

Color	Exercise
Eat healthy	Get enough sleep
Hug a loved one	Nature walk
Cook	Quiet time

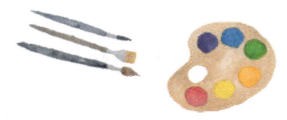

Intentionally left blank for double sided printing

Circle coping skills that are healthy. Put an X on coping skills that are not healthy.

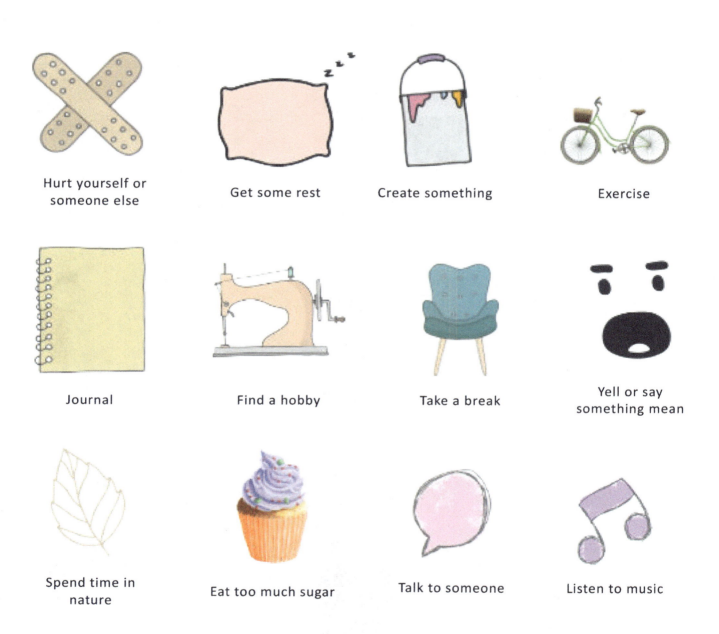

Hurt yourself or someone else	Get some rest	Create something	Exercise
Journal	Find a hobby	Take a break	Yell or say something mean
Spend time in nature	Eat too much sugar	Talk to someone	Listen to music

How do your decisions honor God? Are they helpful or harmful to your mental health and to the health of those around you? Is there anything you need to improve? What have you been doing well?

More coping skills! Circle the ones that you enjoy.

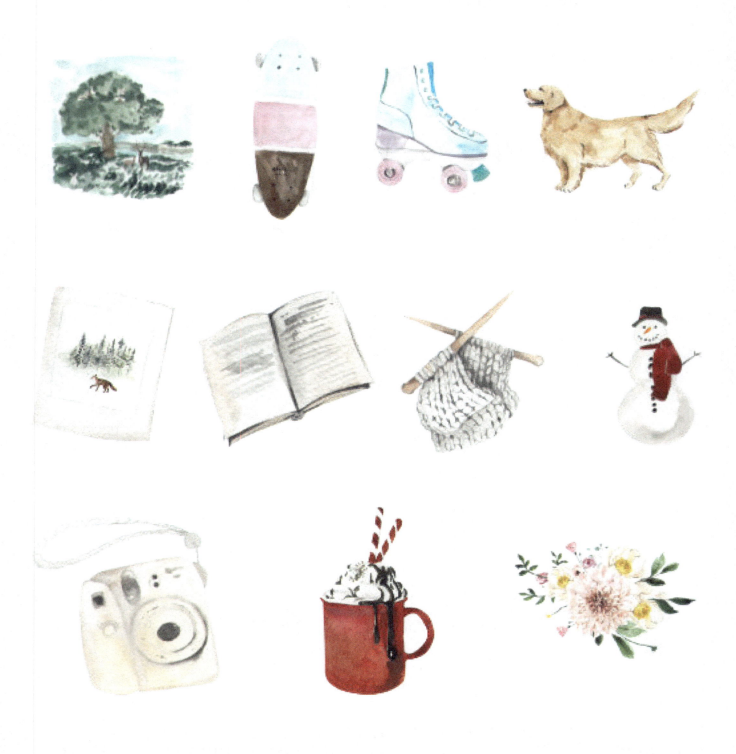

Spending time outside is a fantastic way to improve your mental health. Circle the activities you enjoy doing the most!

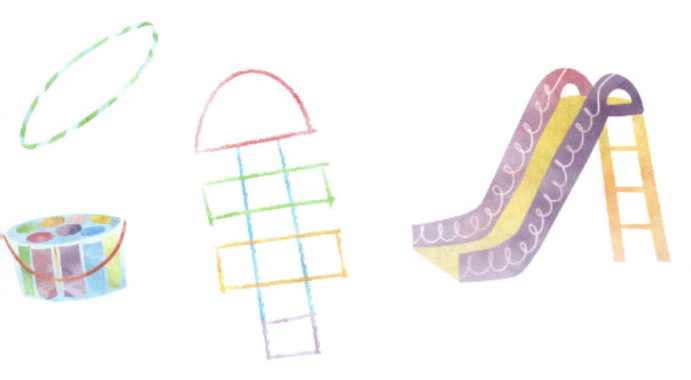

Creativity is another great way to improve your mood! What's your favorite way to be creative?

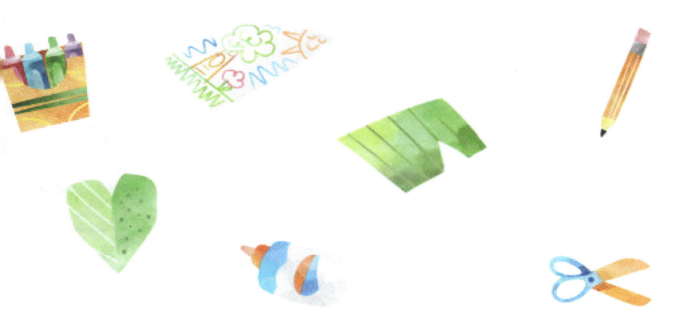

More coping skills! Circle the ones you enjoy. Make a list of the ones that are the most helpful to you.

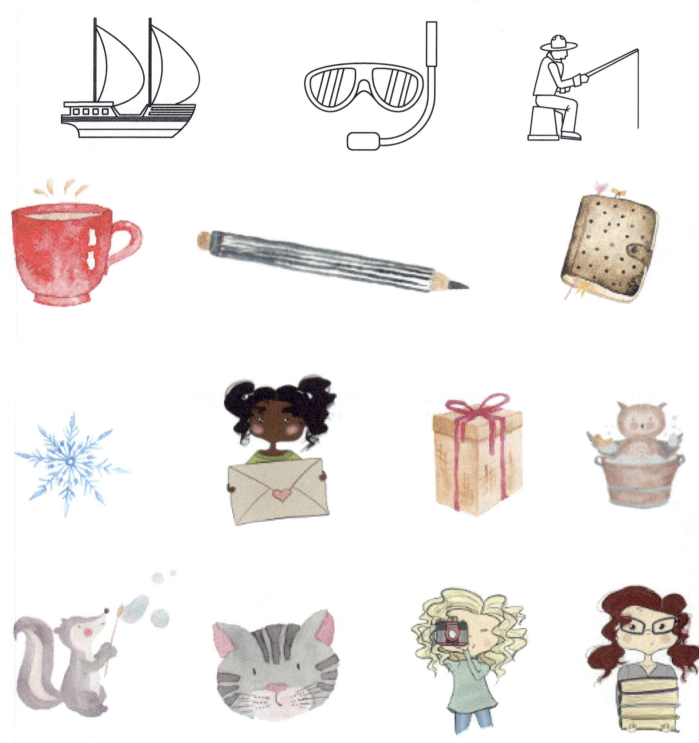

Coping Skills
Complete the crossword puzzle below

Name:_____

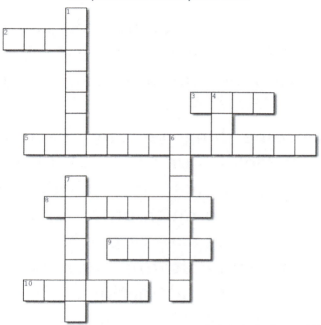

Across
2. when you talk to God
3. tell someone about your problems
5. how we can use our lungs to calm down
8. when we protect our personal or emotional space
9. listening to this can help us calm down
10. when you worship God

Down
1. when you keep your body and clothes clean
4. being creative
6. physical activity that helps us feel better
7. write out your thoughts and feelings

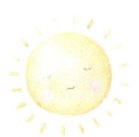

Unhealthy Coping Skills

Did you know that coping skills can also be unhealthy? We may do things that we don't even realize are unhelpful or actually hurting us!

Here are some things we should avoid doing:
Stuffing our feelings or denying that we feel bad
Eating too much or not enough
Sleeping too much or not enough
Stop taking care of our hygiene
Not communicating our needs
Procrastinating
Blaming others for our behavior
Being critical of others
Not asking for help
Not setting healthy boundaries
Bullying others
Being overly critical of ourselves or others
Refusing to ask for help
Isolating

Can you think of any others? Discuss with your loved one why these behaviors are unhelpful and what you can do instead. Remember, it's okay to ask for help!

Let's practice improving our focus. When we are aware of our environment, we can cope more effectively with hard feelings such as anger or anxiety. For each word, find something that describes it:

Blue
Yellow
White
Purple
Small
Tall
Circle
Hot
Hard
Loud

Red
Green
Black
Orange
Big
Short
Square
Cold
Soft
Quiet

Where is my focus? On my problems or on God? We can get caught up in being sad or worried about things in our past and future. When we focus on eternity with God, our perspective and mood will change.

Hymn: Turn Your Eyes Upon Jesus

"Keep your eyes focused on what is right. Keep looking straight ahead to what is good." Hebrews 12:2

More exercises to improve our focus:

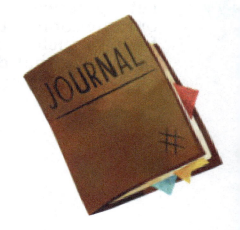

Create something using blocks or clay
Complete a puzzle
Complete a word search or crossword puzzle
Color or paint
Sew/crochet
Games: I Spy, Simon Says, Freeze Dance

Choose one and then journal your thoughts/feelings about the activity here:

_____

_____

_____

_____

Nature Scavenger Hunt

This exercise can improve our focus and encourage us to spend time in God's creation, both of which will help improve our mood! See if you can find the following things in nature.

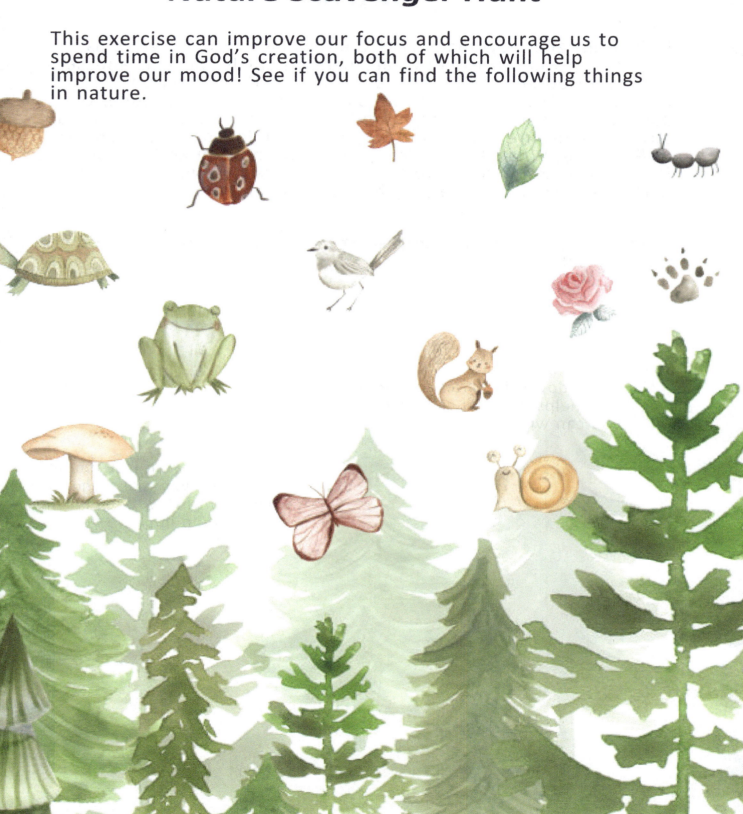

Music

Isn't it amazing how many gifts God has given us? He gives us glimpses of Heaven while we are here on Earth. Music is another gift from God and it can have a powerful influence on our emotions. Notice the lyrics, the background music, the tone, the pauses, the silence. The right kind of music can help decrease our stress. Hymns are a beautiful way to be reminded of the richness of Scripture. What do you like to listen to in order to feel calm? Do the lyrics remind you to honor God? (Classical music can be particularly soothing and may help with sleep!)

Older children may want to research the benefits music has on our mental health.

Write down the lyrics to a song that helps you feel calm. Or you can write your own!

Do you play an instrument? You can even make one of your own! How does playing music help improve your mood?

Spend some time listening to various instruments and types of music. Notice how you feel listening to each one. Which ones help you feel calm? Happy? Joyful? How can you use music to help you cope with stress? Circle the instruments you enjoy the most.

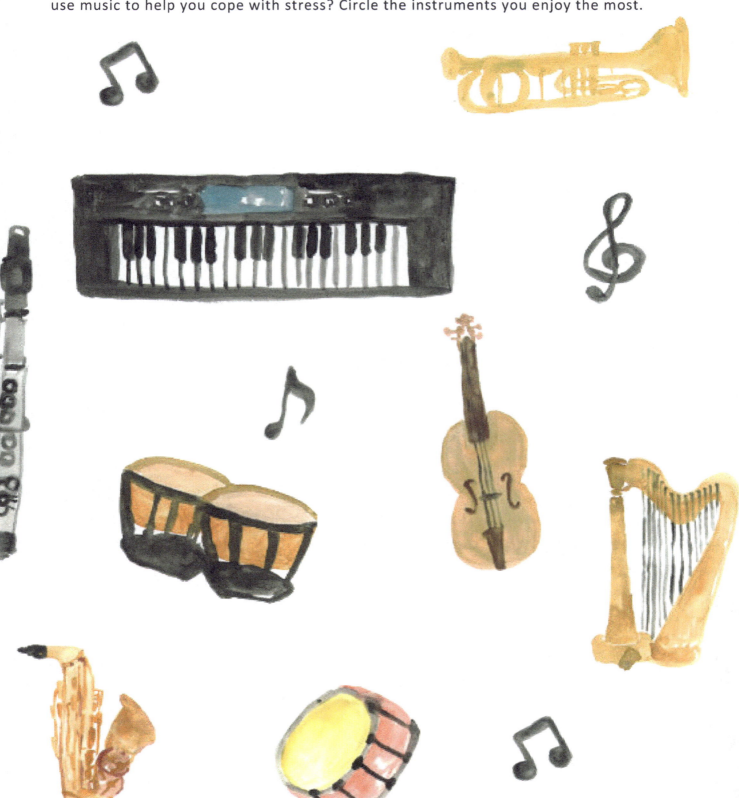

Music

Name 3 songs that make you feel happy.

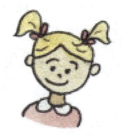

Name 3 songs that are energizing and uplifting.

Name 3 songs that help you relax and feel peaceful.

Name 3 songs that help you feel closer to God.

Copy the following Bible verse. See if you can memorize it!

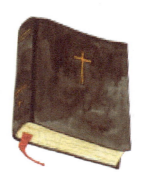

"Sing praises to the Lord. Praise our God with harps." Psalm 147:7 (ICB)

_____

_____

_____

_____

What's your favorite Christian song or hymn? Write down the lyrics here and then try to find them in the Bible. What Bible verses are referenced in the song and how can you use them in your life right now?

_____

_____

_____

_____

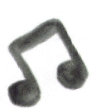
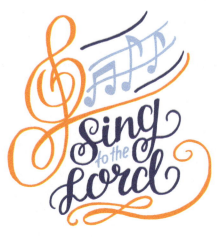

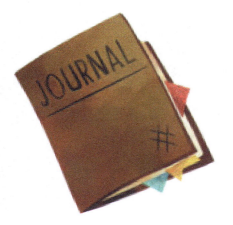

Using the song and Bible verses from the previous page, journal what you learned or felt. Or you can use this page to write your own song of praise to our Lord! You can also write a poem or a prayer. Remember, God cares more about what's in our heart than the words we use to communicate with Him.

_____

_____

_____

_____

Take some time to write or draw your thoughts about this chapter. Use the reflection questions on the next page to guide you!

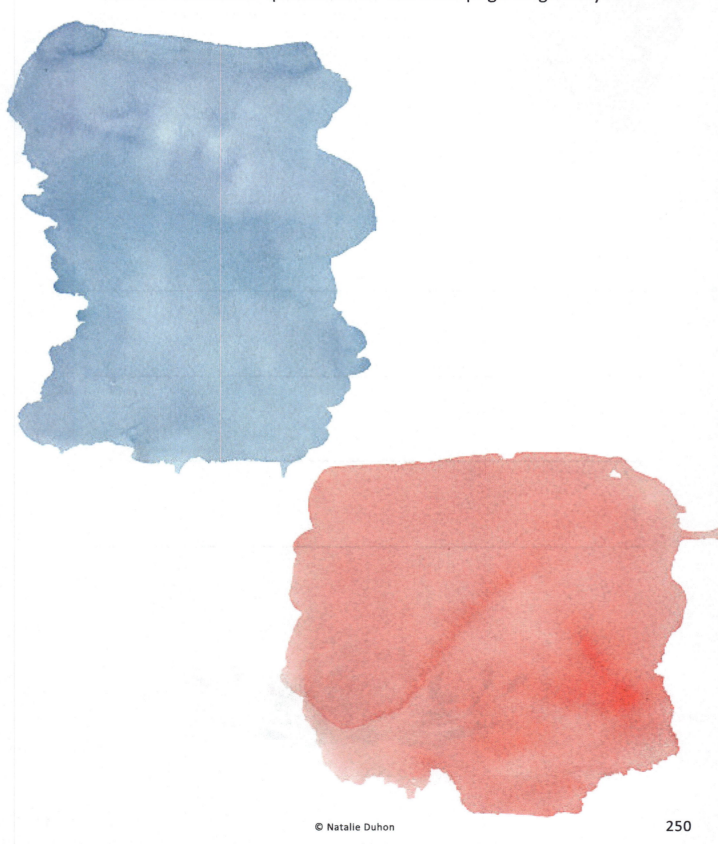

© Natalie Duhon

Reflection

What did you learn about coping skills? How did this lesson add to the knowledge you already had about coping skills?
What questions do you still have?
What are some unhealthy coping skills you need to stop doing? What can you replace them with?
Which exercise in this lesson was the most beneficial to you?

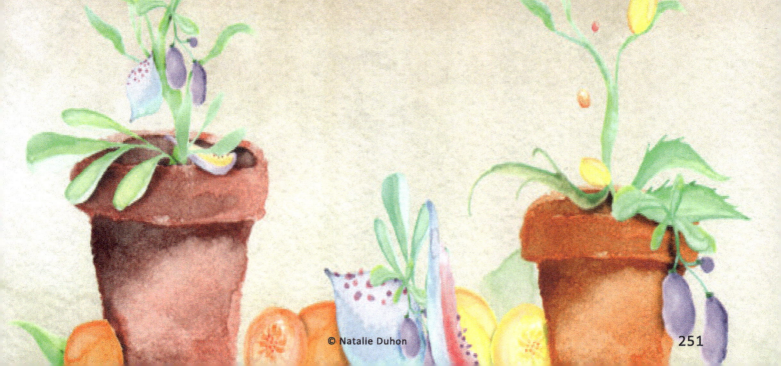

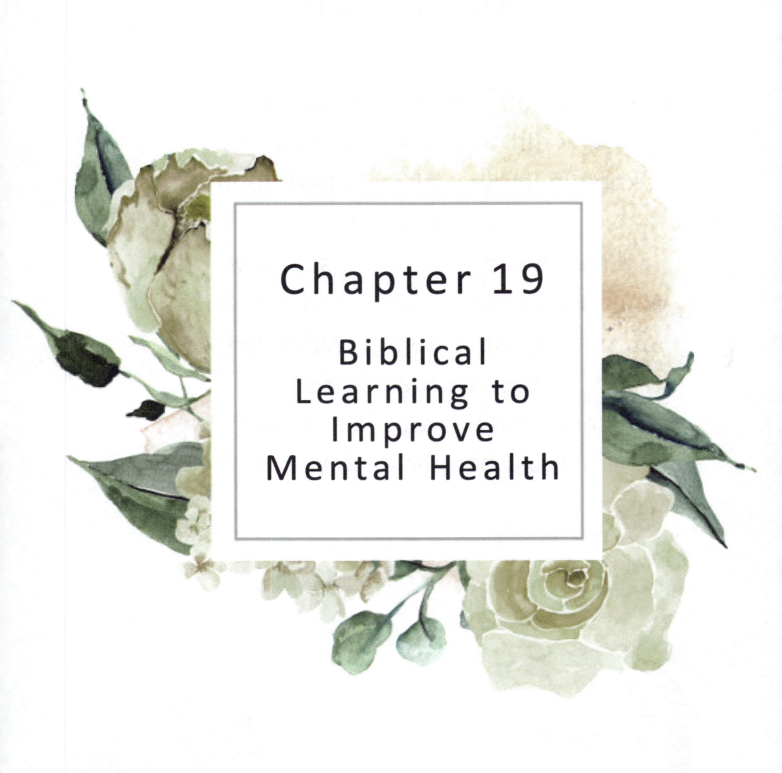

Draw yourself wearing the armor of God.

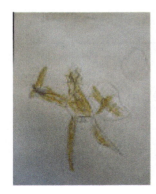 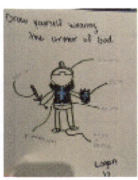 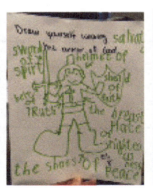 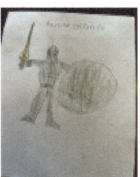

Micah-age 5   Logan-age 12   Eli-age 8   Elijah-age 8

"Finally, be strong in the Lord and in His great power. Wear the full armor of God. Wear God's armor so that you can fight against the devil's evil tricks. Our fight is not against people on earth. We are fighting against the rulers and authorities and the powers of this world's darkness. We are fighting against the spiritual powers of evil in the heavenly world. That is why you need to get God's full armor. Then on the day of evil you will be able to stand strong. And when you have finished the whole fight, you will still be standing. So stand strong, with the belt of truth tied around your waist. And on your chest wear the protection of right living. And on your feet wear the Good News of peace to help you stand strong. And also use the shield of faith. With that you can stop all the burning arrows of the Evil One. Accept God's salvation to be your helmet. And take the sword of the Spirit—that sword is the teaching of God. Pray in the Spirit at all times. Pray with all kinds of prayers, and ask for everything you need. To do this you must always be ready. Never give up. Always pray for all God's people." Ephesians 6:10-18 (ICB)

How have I shown these fruits in my life? Which ones do I need to improve? Ask a loved one for their honest input.

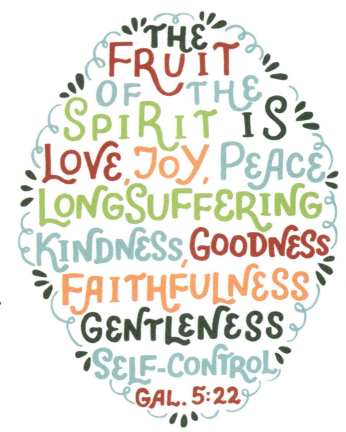

Write down a prayer to ask for God's grace.

_____

_____

_____

_____

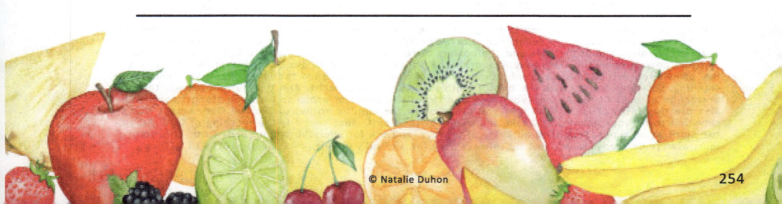

Have you ever had to wait patiently when you really wanted something? Maybe it was something simple, like dessert. Or maybe you had to wait patiently for something really important. How can we focus on God while waiting patiently on Him?

"Patience is better than strength. Controlling your temper is better than capturing a city." Proverbs 16:32 (ICB)

Sometimes we expect God to answer our prayers right away. This isn't always how God works and sometimes we have to wait a long time to receive an answer. Does this mean He isn't listening? Of course not! The Bible assures us God always hears our prayers. Think about the stories we read in the Bible. They're all true! But what we read in a paragraph or two may have taken place over years, decades, or even centuries! These were real people who trusted God even though they didn't understand what was going on at the time. We don't always understand God's plan right away. However, the Bible shows us repeatedly that we can trust Him.

Psalm 22:24 (ICB) says, **"The Lord does not ignore the one who is in trouble. He doesn't hide from him. He listens when the one in trouble calls out to Him."**

In Jeremiah 29:11 (ICB), we read, **"I say this because I know what I have planned for you,"** says the Lord. **"I have good plans for you. I don't plan to hurt you. I plan to give you hope and a good future."**

Self-control

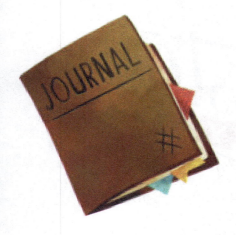

In what areas of my life do I need to work on self-control? How can I use what I have learned so far to improve my self-control? Do I need to work on waiting my turn? Do I need to take a deep breath before I say something mean? Maybe I need to remind myself to choose gratitude instead of complaining. Remember, we are a work in progress and can always ask God for His help! Journal your thoughts here.

_____

_____

_____

_____

Draw a picture of a tower. How can this picture help you remember this Bible verse? How can this verse bring comfort during difficult times? You can also use blocks or clay to build one!

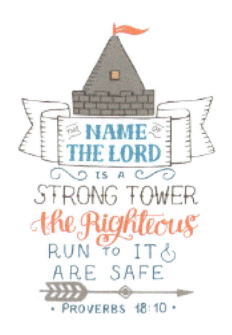

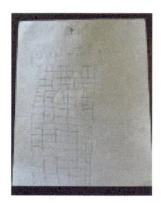

Elijah-age 8

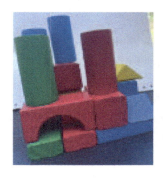

Elizabeth-age 7

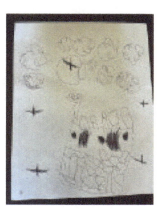

Micah-age 5

"The heavens tell the glory of God. And the skies announce what His hands have made. Day after day they tell the story. Night after night they tell it again. They have no speech or words. They don't make any sound to be heard. But their message goes out through all the world. It goes everywhere on Earth. The sky is like a home for the sun."
Psalm 19:1-4 (ICB)

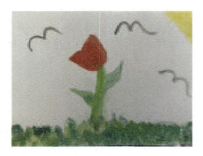

Nicole-age 11

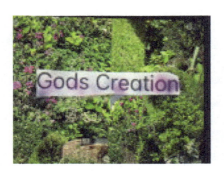

Nicole-age 11

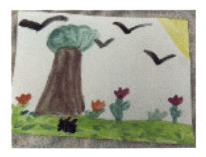

Candace- age 7

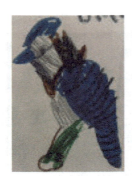

Elizabeth- age 7

Draw something in God's creation that brings you joy. Say a prayer thanking God for this part of His creation. How can you be more intentional about noticing His creation and thanking God for what He has made for us? God's creation helps us recognize His power and glory. We can't help but feel grateful when we think about what God has given us.

© Natalie Duhon

Name:_____

God's Creation

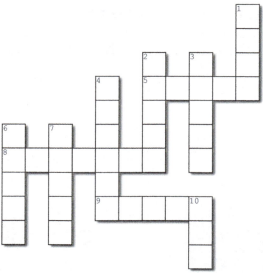

Across
5. the planet we live on
8. creatures created on the sixth day
9. you see them when you up at the nighttime sky

Down
1. they swim in the ocean
2. what a plant or tree grows from
3. green and grows from the ground
4. Adam was the first, Eve was the second
6. liquid we need to survive
7. animals that fly
10. gives Earth light and heat

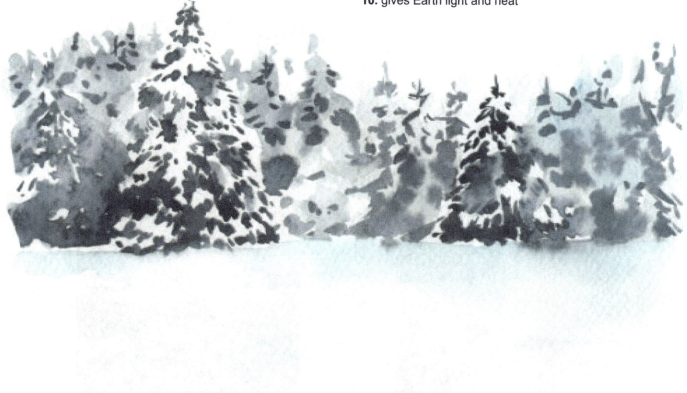

Describe the four seasons that God created. Write down or draw two things in each season that brings you joy. You can also research what's unique about each season where you live. How does seeing the beauty in God's creation impact your mood? The consistency of the seasons each year reminds us of the faithfulness of our God.

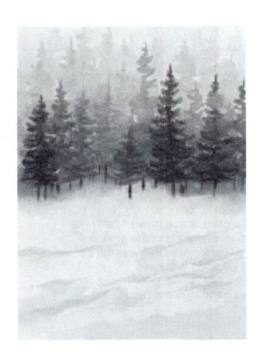
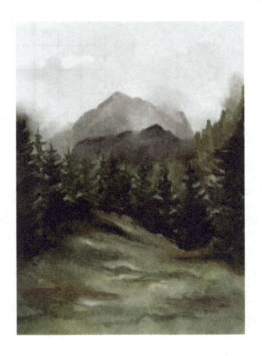
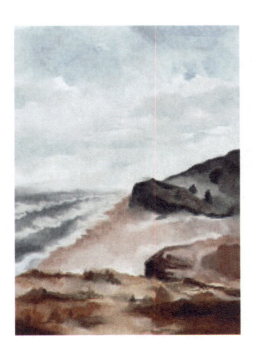
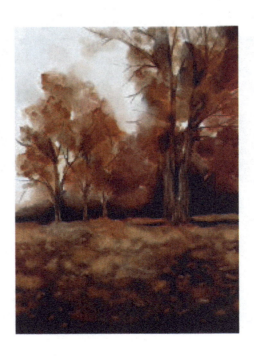

Write a timeline of your life. Ask a loved one to help you start at the very beginning. Where have you seen God's blessings in your life so far?

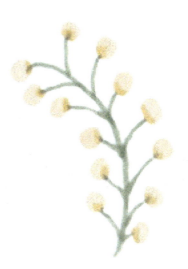

Draw a picture for each day of creation. If God is powerful enough to create the world, He is powerful enough to help me with my struggles. Pray to God now, to thank Him for what He has done in the past and what He promises to do in the future.

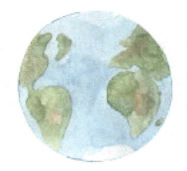

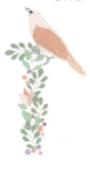  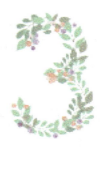 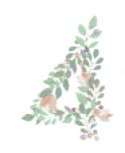

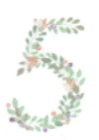 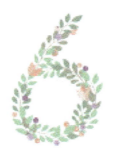 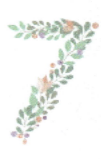

Find five beautiful things that God created. Spend some time drawing/painting them, writing about them, or taking pictures of them to make a collage. Or you can collect various things in nature and make a nature collage. Notice the colors, shapes, and patterns you see in nature. Say a prayer of thanks to God for His creation.

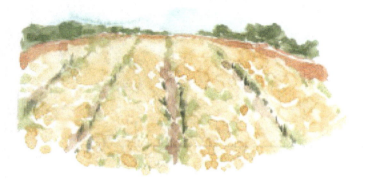

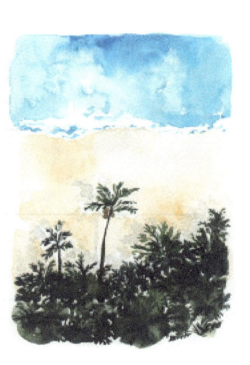

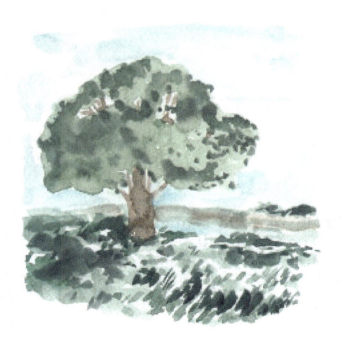

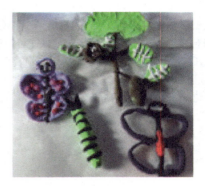

Elizabeth-age 7

Think about how a caterpillar has to go through many changes to transform into a butterfly. Draw a butterfly on a separate sheet of paper and decorate it with glitter, tissue paper, sequins, or something else. Or you can make one out of clay. Be creative! Then write about how you can be transformed or grow in your faith.

_____

_____

_____

_____

"Do not be shaped by this world. Instead be changed within by a new way of thinking. Then you will be able to decide what God wants for you. And you will be able to know what is good and pleasing to God and what is perfect."   Romans 12:2 (ICB)

Pick two people in the Bible who overcame adversity and never gave up. (One example is in the book of Ruth). Write down in your own words how they overcame their struggles. What did you learn that can help you cope with your current struggles?

"Then God will strengthen you with His own great power. And you will not give up when troubles come, but you will be patient." Colossians 1:11 (ICB)

_____

_____

_____

_____

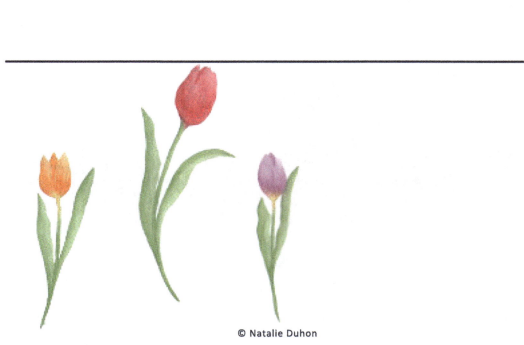

Find two Bible verses that provide you comfort and write them down. Share them with a loved one and share why you chose them. Pick one to memorize.

_____

_____

_____

_____

Pick a person in the Bible who inspires you.
What traits do they have that inspire you?
Which of these traits do you share?

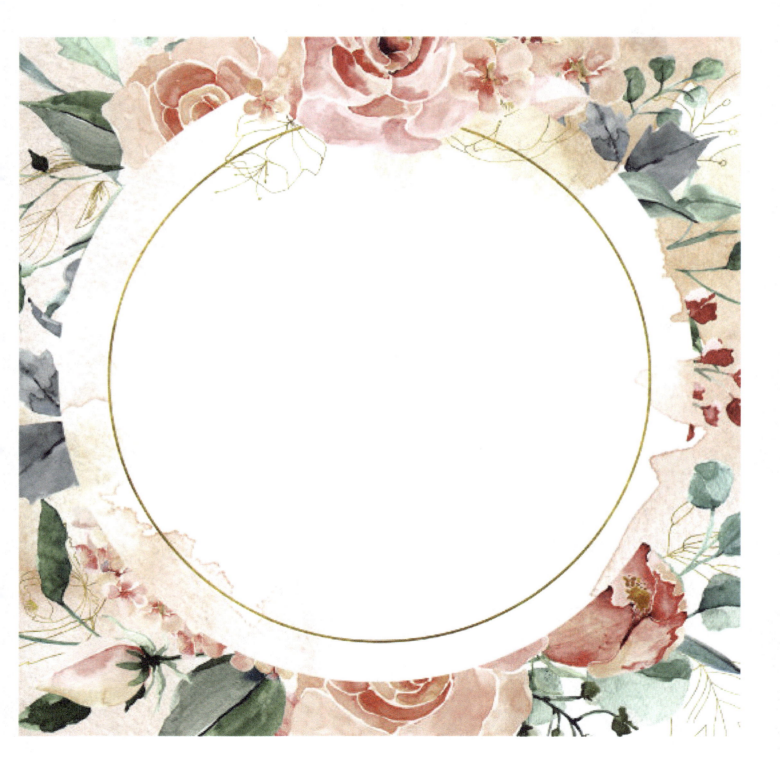

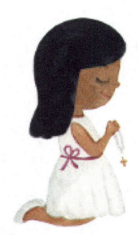

Draw or write about someone you would like to pray for. Spend a few minutes in prayer for that person. How does praying for someone else impact your mood? How can cultivating a habit of prayer improve your mental health?

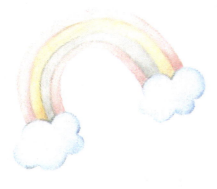

Draw a rainbow. What promise does it signify? What other promises from God can you lean on in times of struggle?

Choose one of God's promises that you can lean on in times of struggle and write it here:

_____

_____

Bible scavenger hunt: Find a person in the Bible who demonstrated these traits:

Strength	Trust
Patience	Wisdom
Faith	Joy
Forgiveness	Peace
Encouragement	Perseverance
Self-control	Courage
Obedience	Mercy
Generosity	Kindness
Love	Compassion

When have you demonstrated some of these traits? When have you witnessed a loved one demonstrate them? Say a prayer asking God to help you develop/improve these traits.

Bible scavenger hunt: Find a person in the Bible who demonstrated these traits and discuss their consequences:

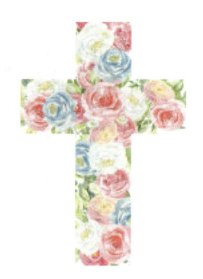

Jealousy

Greed/Selfishness

Hate

Anger
(other than righteous anger)

Dishonesty

Stubbornness

Impatience

Impulsivity

Carelessness

Laziness

Journal your thoughts about the two Bible scavenger hunts you just completed. What did you learn?

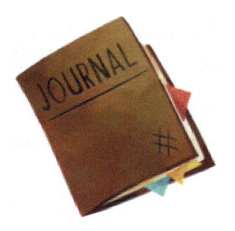

_____

_____

_____

_____

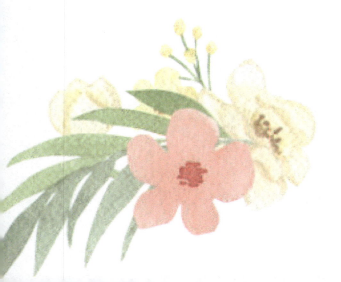

What are the names of God? Which ones give you comfort?

Pick one psalm to memorize and write it here.

_____

_____

_____

_____

"My child, pay attention to my words. Listen closely to what I say. Don't ever forget my words. Keep them deep within your heart. These words are the secret to life for those who find them. They bring health to the whole body."
Proverbs 4:20-22 (ICB)

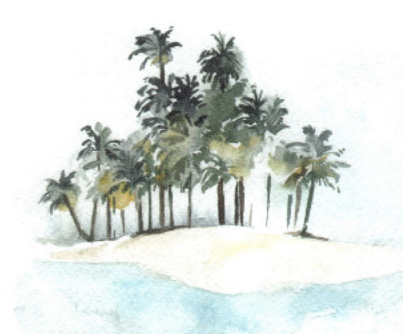

The Ten Commandments

Do you know the 10 commandments? Read Exodus 19-20 and draw or write the 10 commandments here. How do the choices I make honor these commandments? Is there something I need to change?

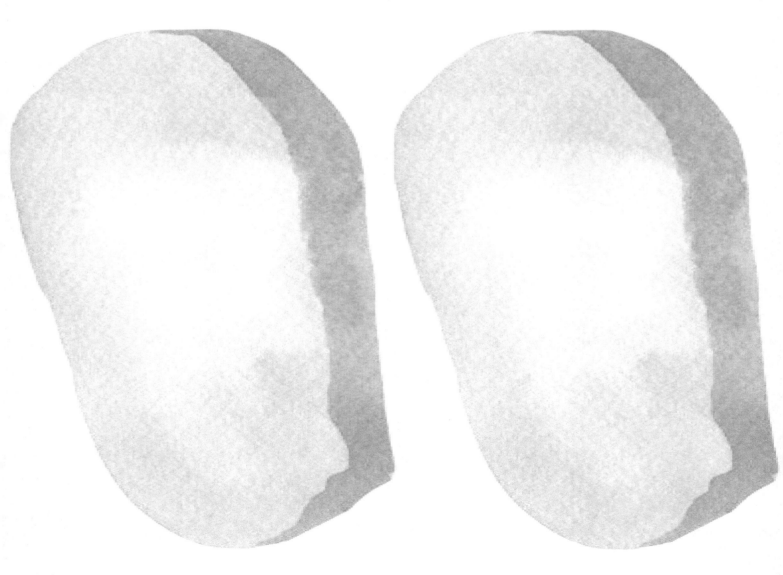

The Sermon on the Mount

Read Matthew 5-7. How can you apply the words of Jesus to your life? How do your choices reflect His teaching?

Psalm 23 (ICB)

"The Lord is my shepherd. I have everything I need. He gives me rest in green pastures. He leads me to calm water. He gives me new strength. For the good of His name, He leads me on paths that are right. Even if I walk through a very dark valley, I will not be afraid because you are with me. Your rod and your shepherd's staff comfort me. You prepare a meal for me in front of my enemies. You pour oil of blessing on my head. You give me more than I can hold. Surely your goodness and love will be with me all my life. And I will live in the house of the Lord forever."

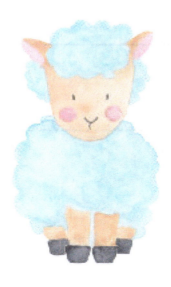

© Natalie Duhon

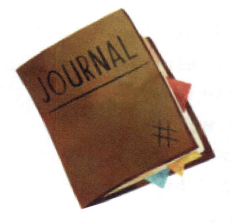

How does Psalm 23 relate to your wants and needs? How can you learn to rely more on God in times of need? How has He provided for you in the past? Journal your thoughts here:

_____

_____

_____

_____

Prayer requests that have been answered (write down dates if possible). This will help us develop gratitude for what we have.

_____

_____

_____

_____

Current prayer requests (write down current date and date prayer is answered). This will help increase our faith and help us be content no matter what. Keep in mind that God's answers don't always look like what we believe they should look like. We can rest assured that God knows best and He has good plans for us.

_____

_____

_____

_____

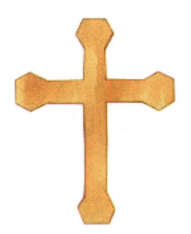

"I will praise you, Lord, with all my heart. I will tell all the miracles you have done."
Psalm 9:1 (ICB)

Read Matthew 7:24-27. Draw yourself building your house on the sand and then building your house on the rock. How does this relate to the choices you make each day? Remember when we discussed goals and habits?

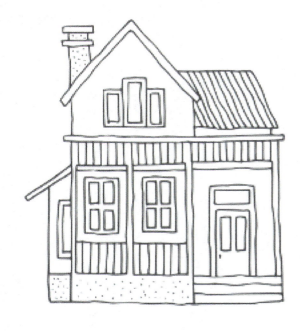

Take some time to write or draw your thoughts about this chapter. Use the reflection questions on the next page to guide you!

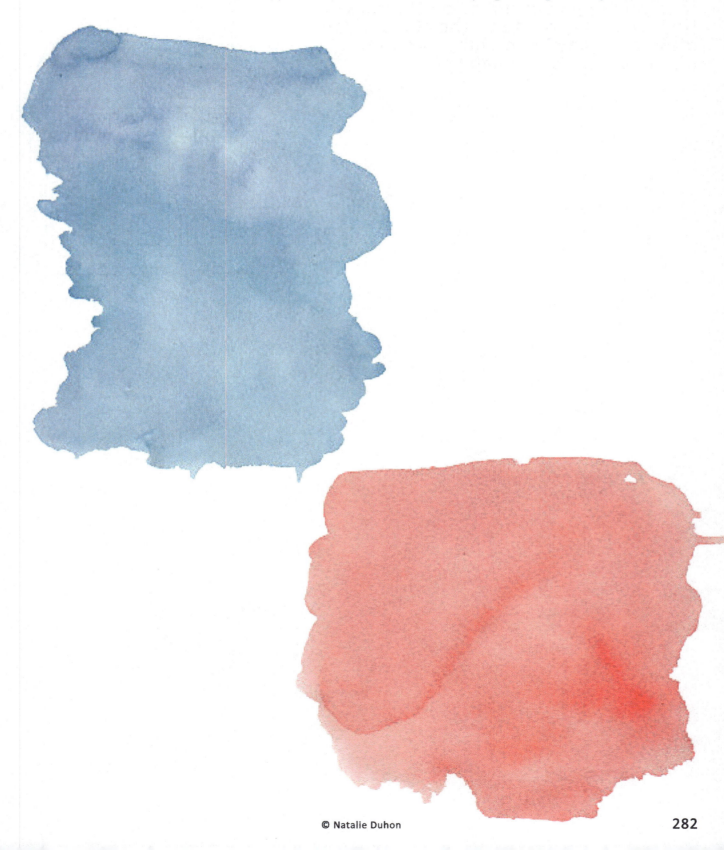

Reflection

Which exercises in this lesson were the most beneficial?

Is there a Bible story that wasn't covered in this lesson that has had a positive impact on you? How can that story help you improve your mental health?

How does reading the Bible consistently help improve your mental health?

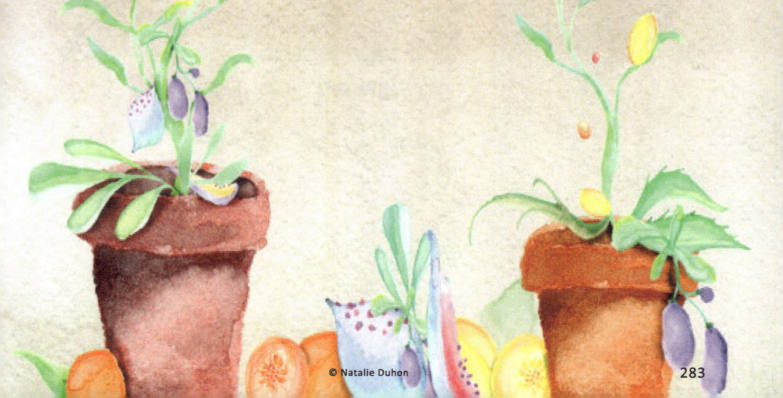

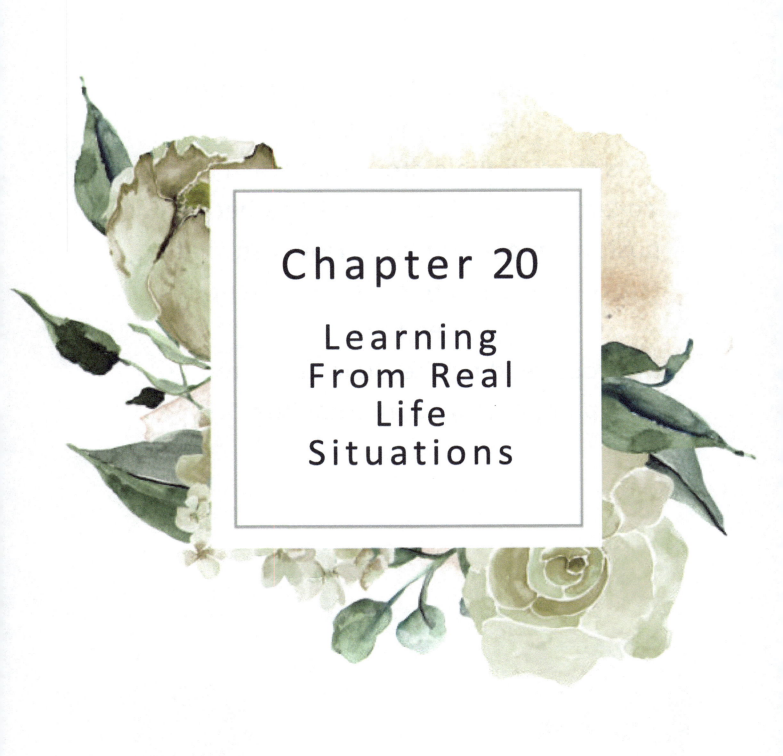

Chapter 20

Learning From Real Life Situations

We've learned a lot so far! Let's explore some real life situations and you can discuss what would be a helpful response for each one.

Nicole, Candace, and Elizabeth were having fun playing with their toy kitchen. Elizabeth saw that Candace put on her favorite green and orange apron. All of a sudden, Elizabeth started crying and tried to take the apron from Candace. She didn't know how what she was feeling, but she knew it didn't feel good.

Elizabeth was feeling jealous. We all feel jealous sometimes. Jealousy is when we want something that someone else has. The Bible has a lot to say about jealousy. How can I be content with what I do have? What am I grateful for? Write down your thoughts here.

_____

_____

_____

_____

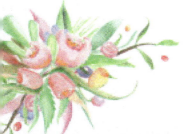

Today we had some friends over to visit. Mommy was holding their friend's baby and all of a sudden, Elizabeth got very upset and wanted Mommy to hold her instead of the baby. Elizabeth was feeling jealous. Even though she knows how much her Mommy loves her, it was hard for her to see her Mommy holding another baby. She felt better when Mommy reassured her and told her how much she loves Elizabeth. We all get jealous sometimes. It helps to talk to someone about how we are feeling. Our trusted adults in our lives can help us learn healthy ways to cope with these hard emotions. Have you ever felt jealous? Write down your thoughts or draw them here.

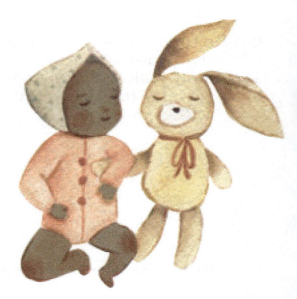

Nicole and Elizabeth were having fun playing in Elizabeth's room while Candace played in the living room. When Elizabeth came to the living room to get a toy, she saw a sad look on Candace's face. Candace had a frown and was looking down at the ground. When Elizabeth asked her what was wrong, Candace told her she felt left out. Elizabeth thought about how she felt when other kids didn't play with her, so she invited Candace to join her and Nicole. The feeling Elizabeth experienced was empathy. Empathy is when we try to imagine how we would feel in a particular situation. This allows us to understand others better and have compassion for them.

Jesus came down from Heaven and experienced life on Earth. He had the same experiences and emotions that we do. Since Jesus has experienced everything we go through, He has empathy for us when we feel bad. Prayer is the most powerful way to cope with our hurt feelings.

When have you shown someone empathy? Share with your loved one.

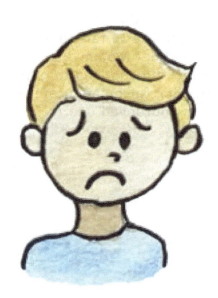

Elizabeth was playing with her friend when her friend's mom had to leave the room for a few minutes. Although Elizabeth's mom was still there, her friend started crying because she missed her mommy. Elizabeth showed empathy and comforted her friend by giving her a hug and telling her "it will be okay." Elizabeth also misses her mommy when she's not around, so she was able to understand how her friend was feeling.

© Natalie Duhon

Last week, Elizabeth had a bad dream. She woke up very scared and ran to her parent's room for comfort. She felt better after she talked to them, but she still worries about the dream. Tonight before bed, she told her Mommy that she felt scared because she didn't want to have another bad dream. She was feeling worried. We all worry sometimes, but the Bible has a lot to teach us about worry! Elizabeth and her Mommy talked about her worries and prayed, asking Jesus for help. They also sang a hymn they learned, Amazing Grace. Prayer, singing, and talking to her Mommy helped Elizabeth feel better.

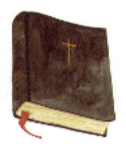 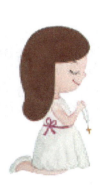 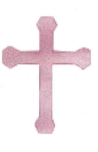

Elizabeth and her parents love to visit Great Grandma in the nursing home. Elizabeth loves to tell Great Grandma about what she's learning in school. Sometimes she feels shy when she goes to the nursing home because so many of the other men and women like to talk to her. She tries to be polite, but sometimes she feels like hiding behind her Mommy. She isn't trying to be rude, and she knows it's important to be respectful and kind to others. She is feeling shy. Her mommy reminded her that learning to communicate with others takes practice. Have you ever felt shy? Discuss with your loved one.

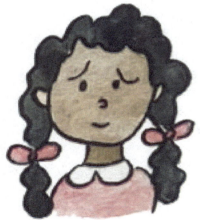

Elizabeth had a rough day at camp. On the way home, Elizabeth said "I want to tell you something, but I'm afraid you'll be mad." Mommy said "I'd rather you be honest with me and we can talk about it." Elizabeth told her Mommy that she was frustrated when her friend cut in front of her, so she pinched her. Mommy told Elizabeth how proud she was that Elizabeth was honest with her. God always wants us to tell the truth, even if it means we may get into trouble. Mommy and Elizabeth had a good conversation and talked about other ways to respond when she gets frustrated.

Do you remember what we learned about anger? There are many ways to describe our anger. They can include frustrated, annoyed, or irritated. What word would you give your anger? What are some good choices we can make when we're angry?

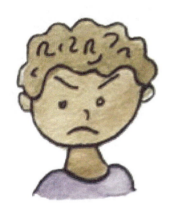

_____

_____

_____

_____

Proverbs 10:9 (ICB) teaches us: "The honest person will live safely. But the one who is dishonest will be caught."

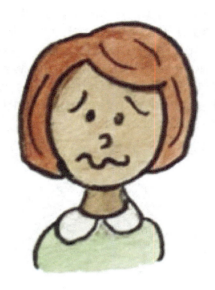

Today Elizabeth got her ears pierced. She had asked her Mommy and Daddy if she could get earrings when she turned five, and she was so excited when they said yes! When the time came to get them pierced, she became very nervous. She was shaking, she had trouble sitting still, and she wanted to run! Her heart was beating fast, her breathing was fast, and she started crying. She was feeling anxious. Her thoughts about the possible pain were worse than the actual pain. Have you ever felt that way? We all get anxious or worried sometimes, but the Bible has a lot to say about what we need to do when we're worried! Draw a picture of yourself coping with your worries in a healthy way.

© Natalie Duhon

Today Aunt Mollie and Uncle Tom came to visit from England. Elizabeth has been looking forward to their trip for months and when they arrived, she ran around the house screeching, jumping around, and hugging them. She is feeling excited!

Draw a picture of something that makes you feel excited.

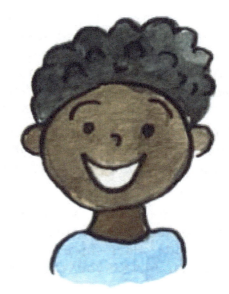

Elizabeth was at the park playing with friends, when she heard someone make a mean comment about another child. At first she froze, not sure what to say or do. She wondered "Should I join in teasing her, so the other kids will like me?" "Should I pretend I didn't hear?" "Should I say something?" "How would I feel if someone said something mean about me?" She also wondered how God would want her to treat others. Wouldn't He want her to treat another person with love?

She continued thinking about the issue and realized that it was important for her to speak up about how it is unkind and unnecessary to tease another human being. She remembered what the Bible said about everyone being made in God's image.

Can you think about a time when you heard someone teasing another person for how they looked, spoke, acted, etc.? What did you do? What could you have done differently? Have you ever teased someone? Have you ever been teased? How did you feel? Journal your thoughts here.

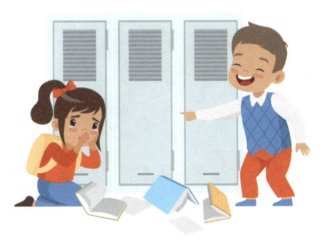

_____

_____

_____

_____

Jacob and Larry wanted to play together, but they couldn't figure out something that they both wanted to do. Jacob wanted to do crafts, while Larry wanted to play with cars. How can they resolve the situation?

Do something different that they both agreed on.
(This is called a compromise).

Other ways to compromise could be:
Play with crafts first, then cars.
Play with cars first, then crafts.

There are many ways we can compromise and make playing with friends a joyful time! Share a time when you had to compromise. Was it easy or hard? How can compromise improve our relationships with others? How can refusing to compromise damage our relationships with others?

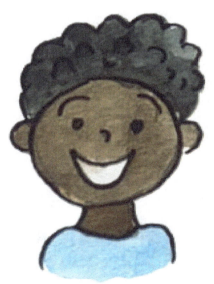

Matthew and Elizabeth were having fun doing arts and crafts with Nana. They were making paper bag puppets and were having fun making all of the different animal sounds! Then Elizabeth told Matthew "Give me the glue!" What's a better way she could have gotten what she wanted?

1. Grabbed the glue from Matthew's hand.

2. Asked Matthew, "Can I please have the glue when you're done with it?"

3. Stopped playing with Matthew because she didn't get what she wanted right away.

4. Started screaming at Matthew.

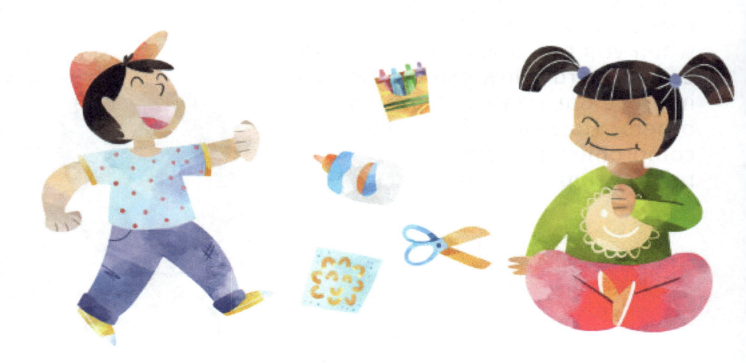

You are playing with a friend and he takes your toy. You quickly became angry and your first thought is to take it back or hit him. Write down two healthy ways you can manage your anger. (Ask a trusted adult for help if needed!)

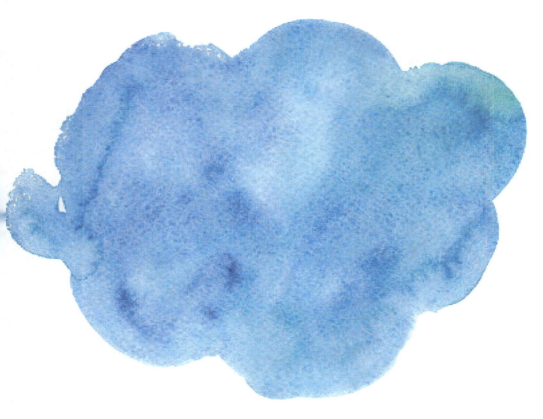

You are playing with a group of friends and one child starts teasing another one. What should you do? Remember what we learned about how we should treat each other?

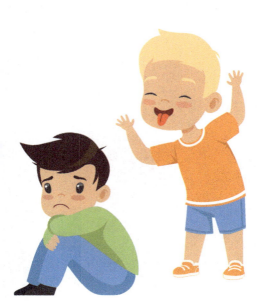

Take some time to write or draw your thoughts about this chapter.
Use the reflection questions on the next page to guide you!

Reflection

What did you learn from the previous situations?
What are some real life situations you've encountered? What did you learn from them? Is there anything you can do differently in the future?
What's been the most impactful thing you've learned from this curriculum? How can it help you moving forward?

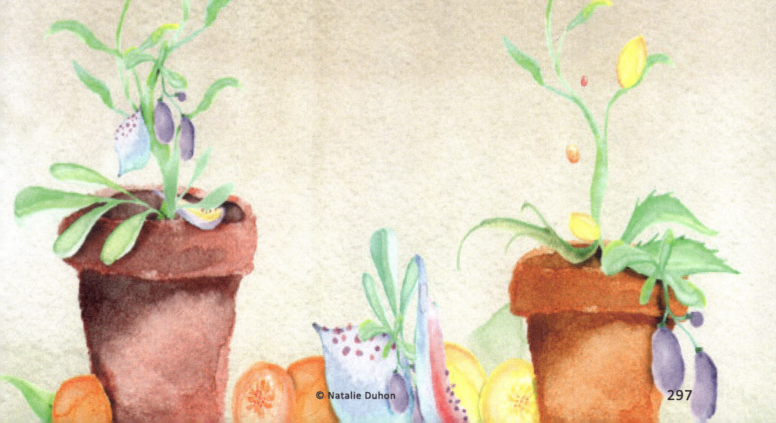

Take some time to explore what you've learned throughout this book. You can revisit the lessons at any time. Use the next few pages to draw or write down some thoughts you have about mental health and everything you have learned. You can also write down any questions you may still have. It's important to be proud of how hard you have worked throughout this book.

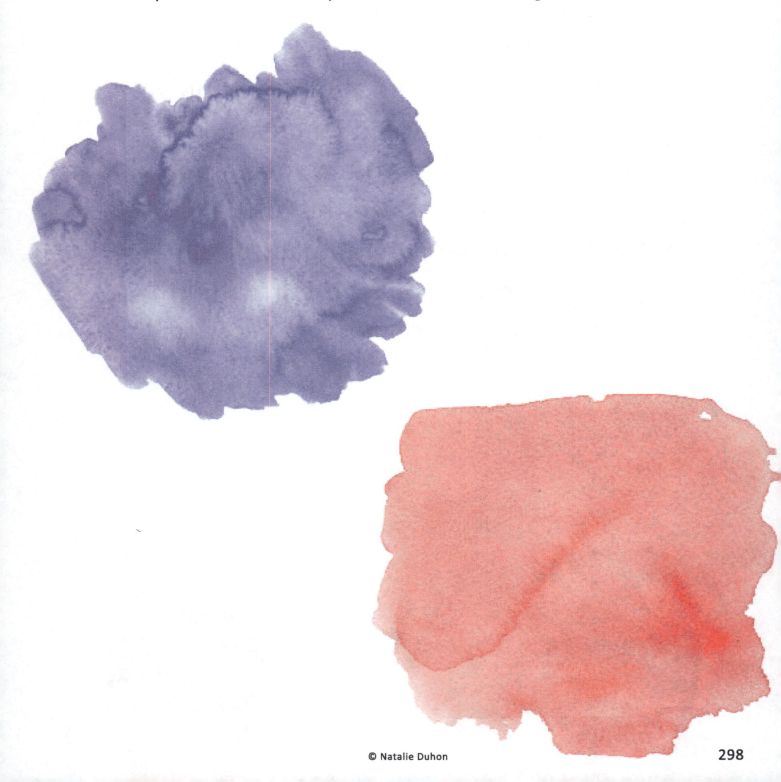

Conclusion

It's important to take the time to reflect on what you and your children have learned. Consider the growth you've both made and what you plan to continue working on. Remember, our mental health is just as important as our physical health. Just as we should eat healthy and exercise regularly, we also want to ensure we are caring for our mental health. Consider revisiting some of the activities at a later time. As your children get older, they will glean more from the information in this book. We are constantly learning about ourselves and about the great God we serve.

Consider reading through your journal again. What have you learned about yourself in the process? What have you learned about the nature of God? Is there someone you feel comfortable sharing your journal with? What steps are you ready to take to continue improving your mental health? How can you continue to guide your child?

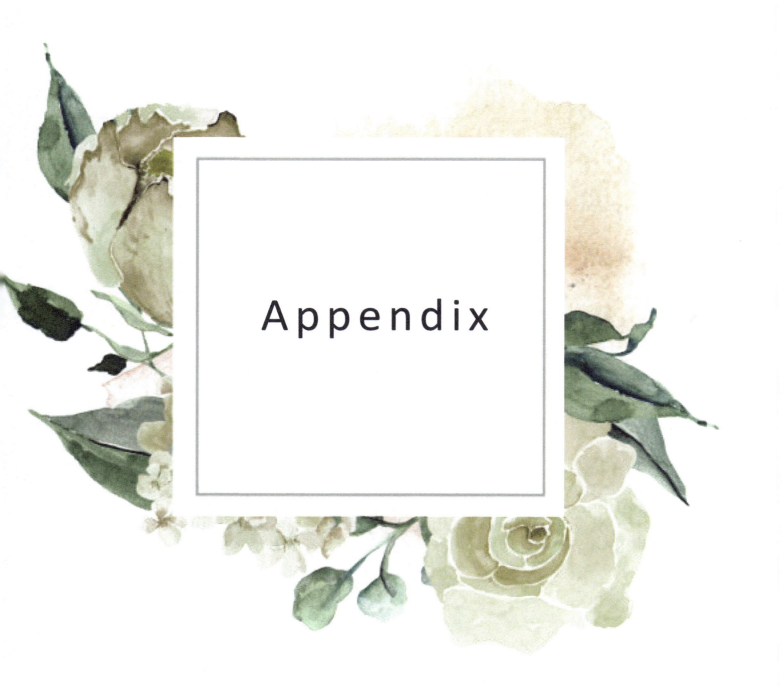

Appendix

Emotion Log

	Morning	Afternoon	Evening
Sunday			
Monday			
Tuesday			
Wednesday			
Thursday			
Friday			
Saturday			

Fill out this emotion log for one week. You may notice that you experience many emotions in one day. Pay attention to any patterns you may see. What did you learn about yourself after doing this exercise?

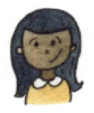 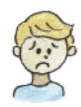 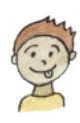 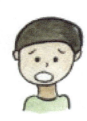

Sample Emotion Log

	Morning	Afternoon	Evening
Sunday	sad	anxious	calm
Monday	happy	happy	happy
Tuesday	angry	sad	sad
Wednesday	anxious	frustrated	excited
Thursday	happy	happy	happy
Friday	happy	happy	happy
Saturday	worried	worried	relaxed

© Natalie Duhon

Name:

Feelings
Complete the crossword puzzle below

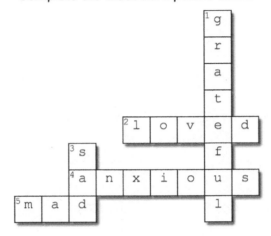

Across
2. when someone cares about us a great deal (**loved**)
4. when we feel worried about something (**anxious**)
5. another word for angry (**mad**)

Down
1. when we appreciate what we have (**grateful**)
3. another word for gloomy (**sad**)

© Natalie Duhon

Name:_____

Coping Skills
Complete the crossword puzzle below

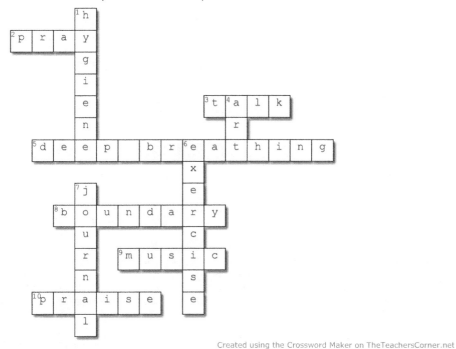

Across
2. when you talk to God (**pray**)
3. tell someone about your problems (**talk**)
5. how we can use our lungs to calm down (**deep breathing**)
8. when we protect our personal or emotional space (**boundary**)
9. listening to this can help us calm down (**music**)
10. when you worship God (**praise**)

Down
1. when you keep your body and clothes clean (**hygiene**)
4. being creative (**art**)
6. physical activity that helps us feel better (**exercise**)
7. write out your thoughts and feelings (**journal**)

© Natalie Duhon

Name:_____

God's Creation

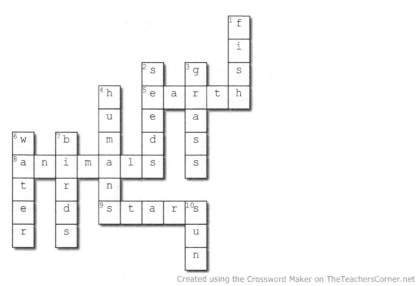

Across
5. the planet we live on (**earth**)
8. creatures created on the sixth day (**animals**)
9. you see them when you up at the nighttime sky (**stars**)

Down
1. they swim in the ocean (**fish**)
2. what a plant or tree grows from (**seeds**)
3. green and grows from the ground (**grass**)
4. Adam was the first, Eve was the second (**humans**)
6. liquid we need to survive (**water**)
7. animals that fly (**birds**)
10. gives Earth light and heat (**sun**)

Anger Iceberg

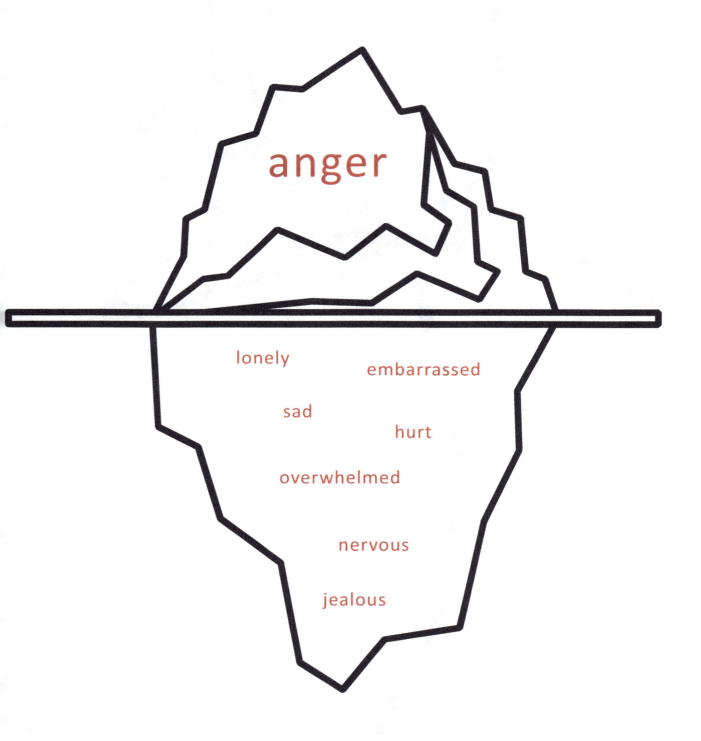

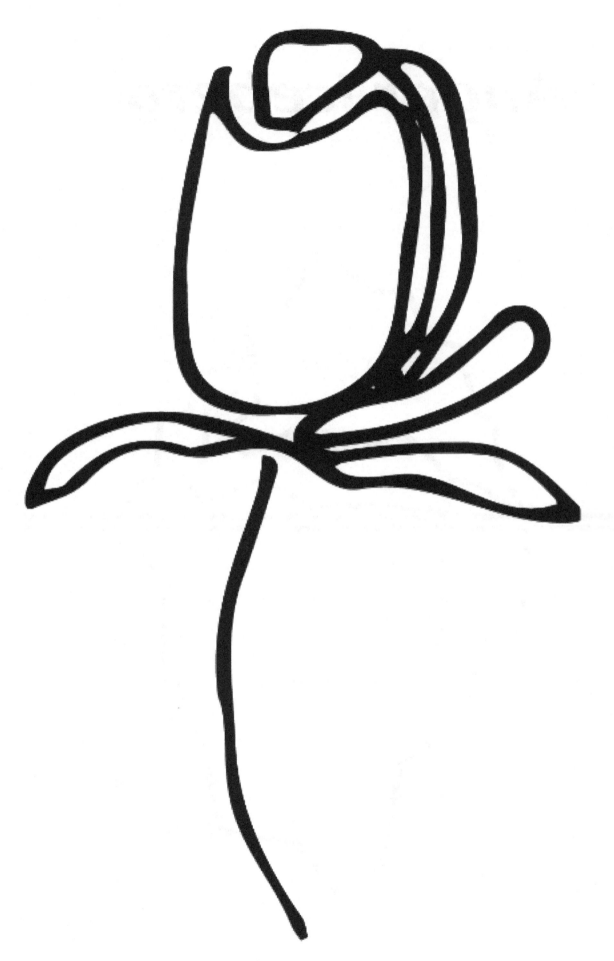

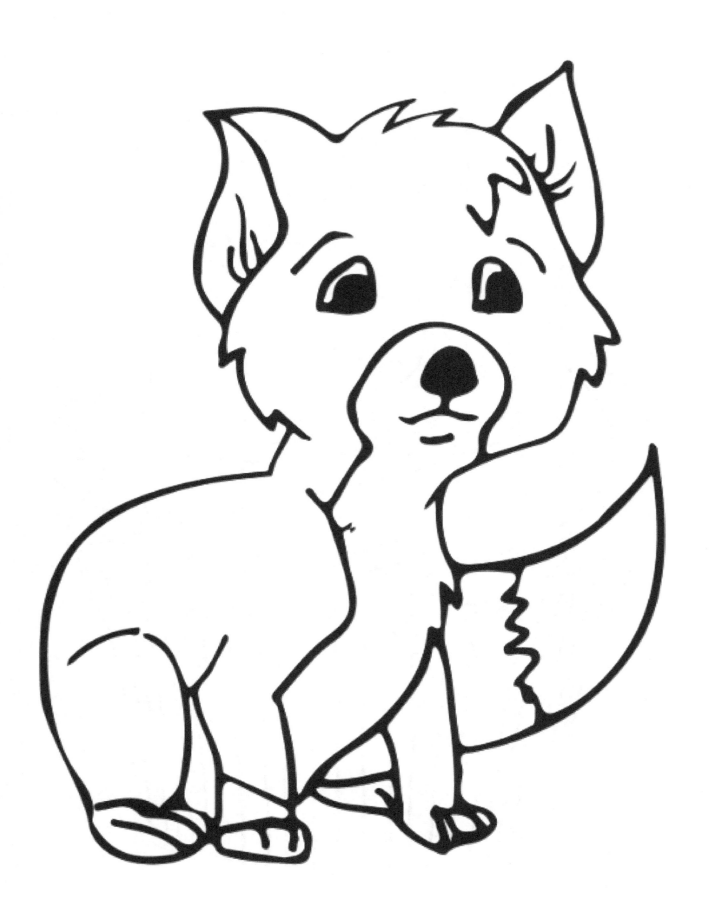

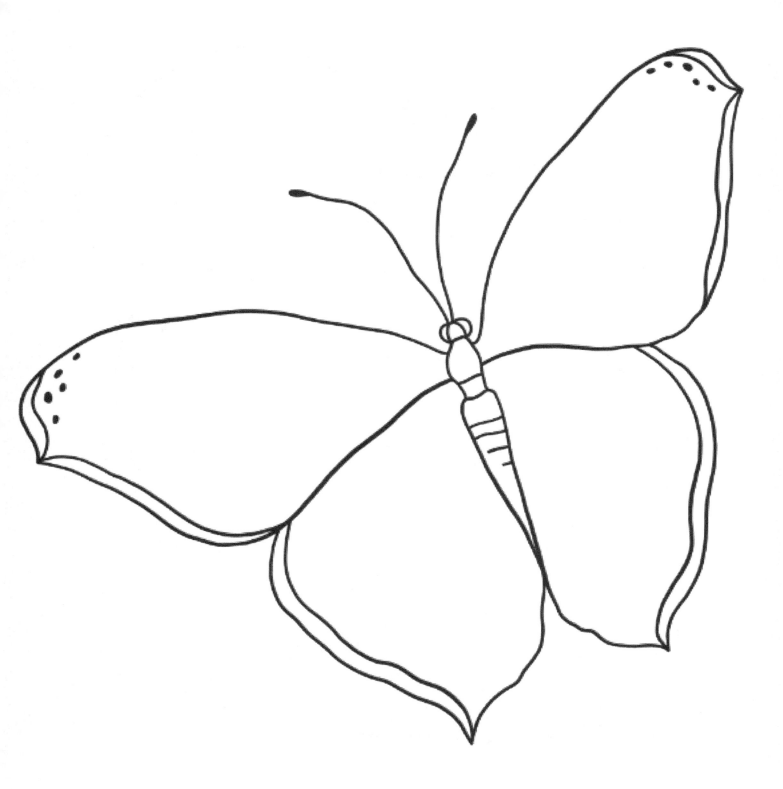

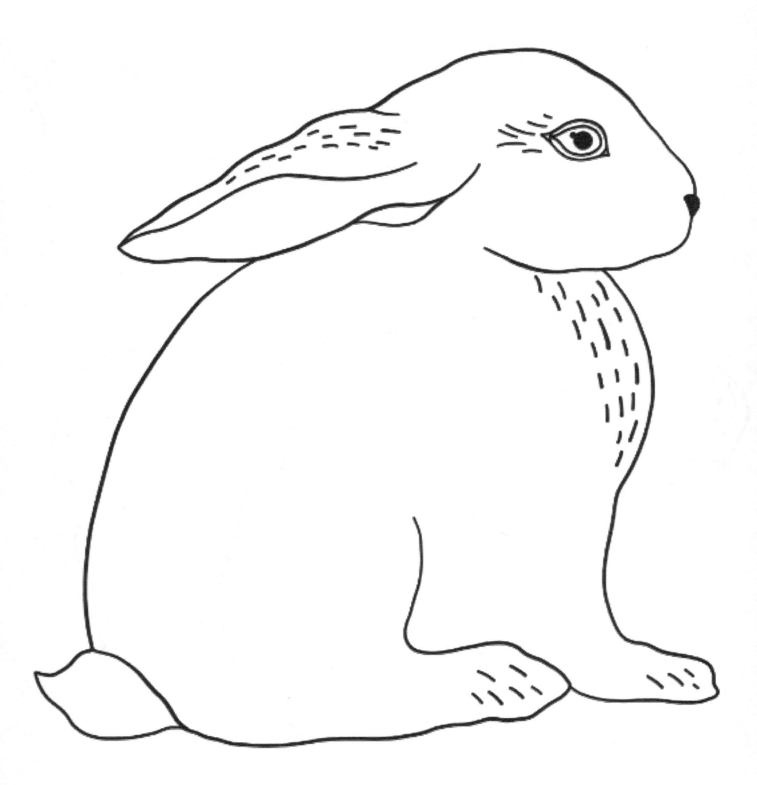

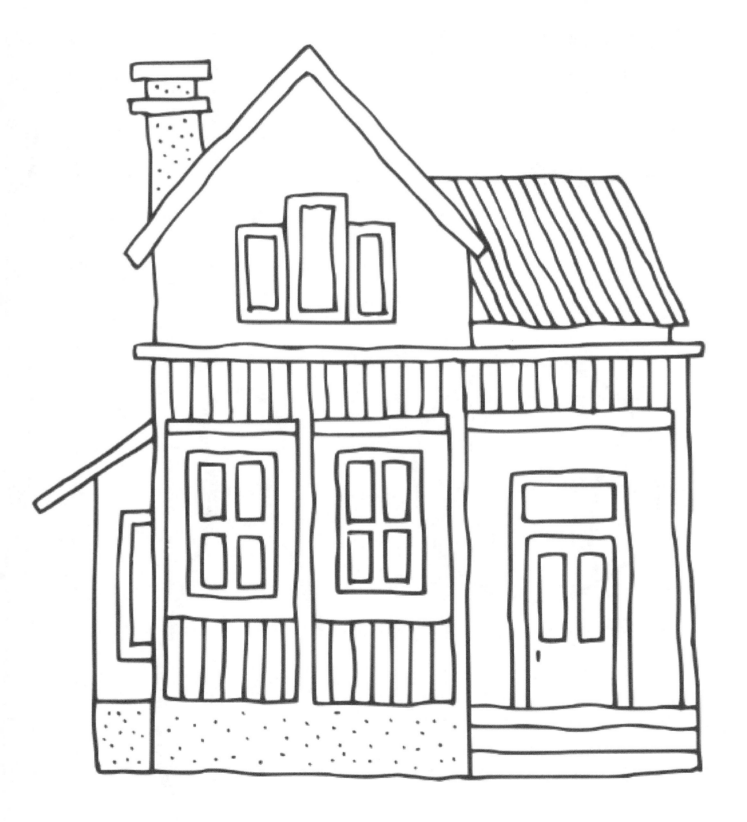

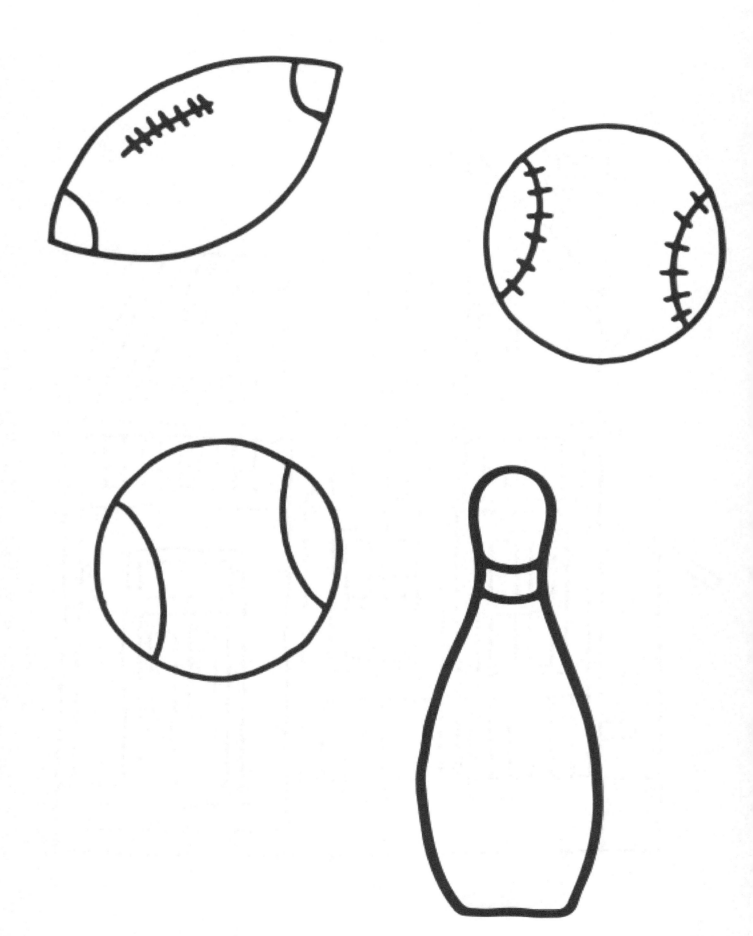

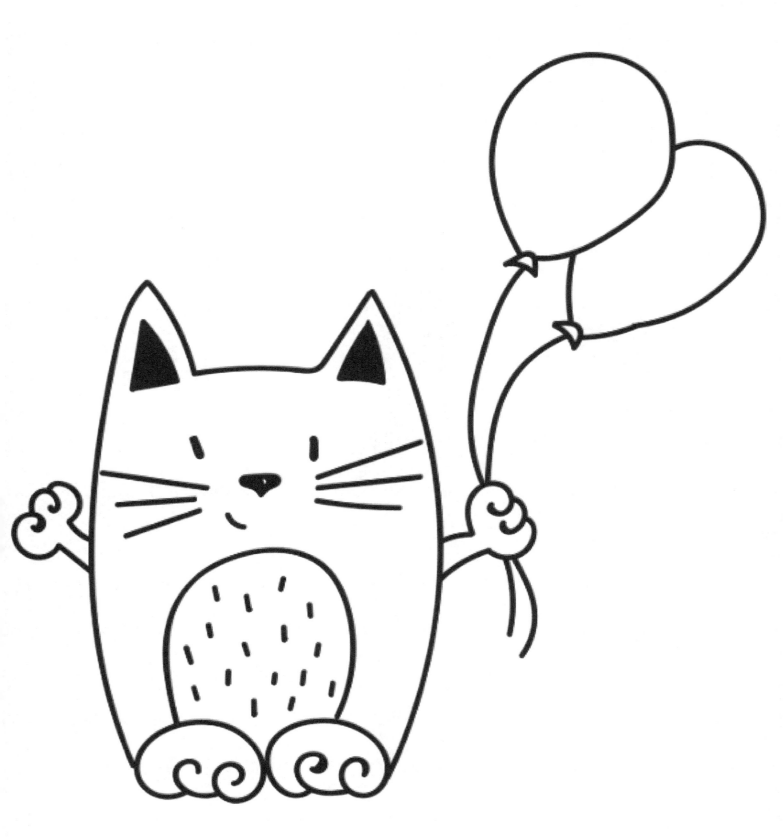

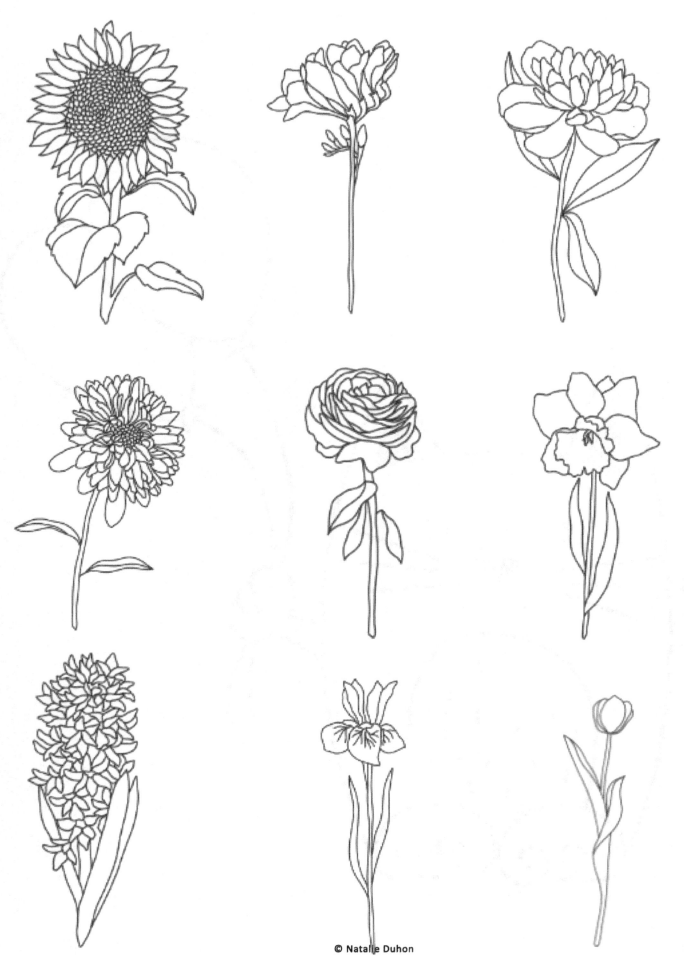

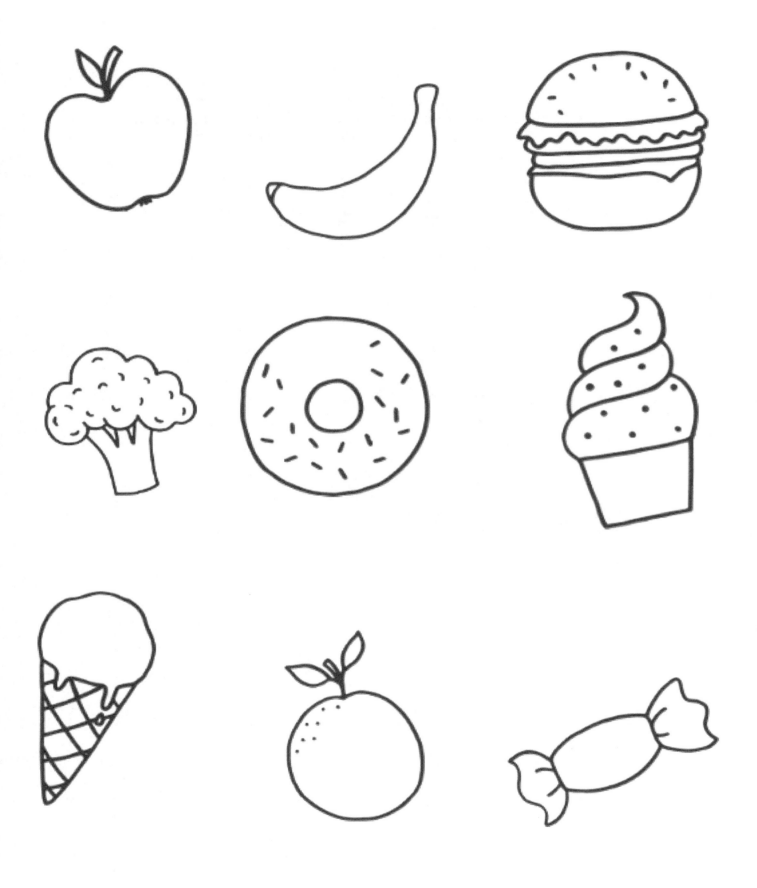

Name the animal! Circle the one that's your favorite. Take a trip to the zoo if you can. How does being in nature and seeing God's creation impact your mood?

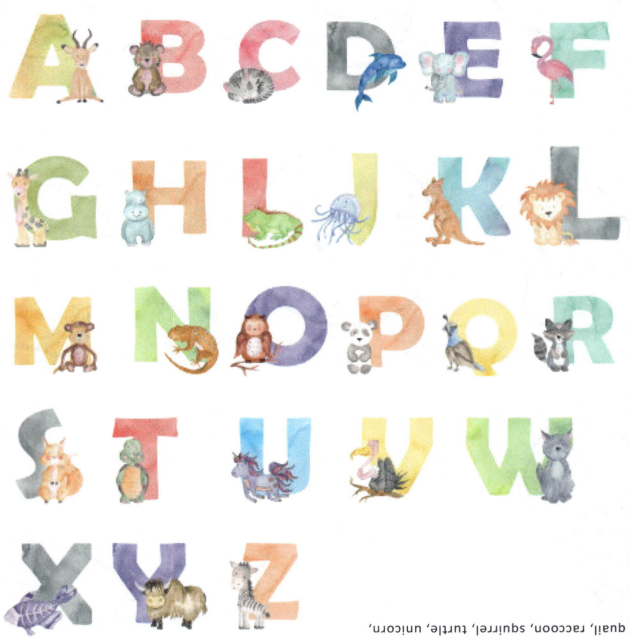

antelope, bear, cat, dolphin, elephant, flamingo, giraffe, hippo, iguana, jelly fish, kangaroo, lion, monkey, newt, owl, panda, quail, raccoon, squirrel, turtle, unicorn, vulture, wolf, x-ray fish, yak, zebra

What's your favorite food? Circle the picture or draw your own!
Can you write the name of each one? Look up the nutritional facts
for some. How can they impact your mental health?

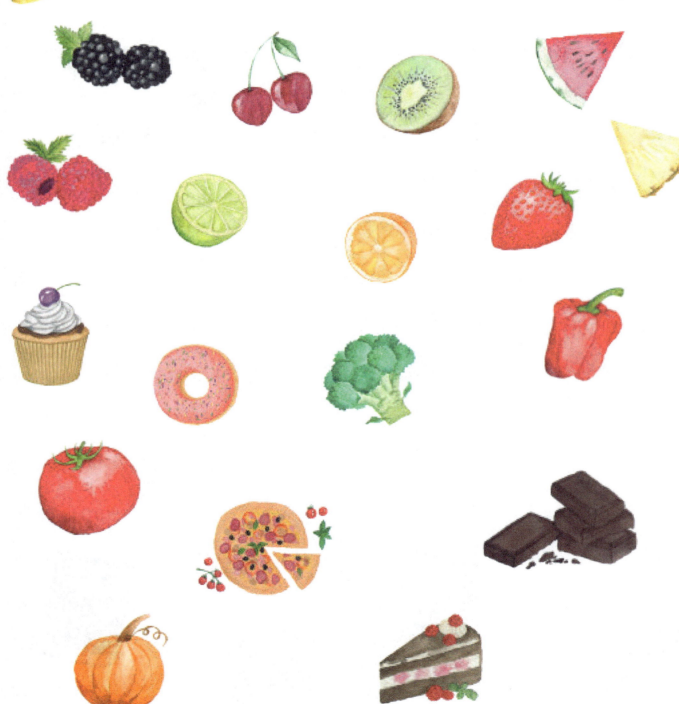

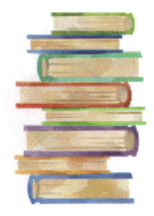

You probably already have some books related to mental health. Write down the ones you have here. Take a trip to the library and find some books about mental health. Use the recommended reading list or pick some of your own!

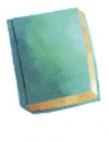
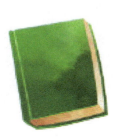
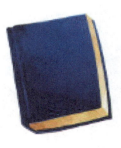

Which parts of the body can you label? Thank God for creating you!

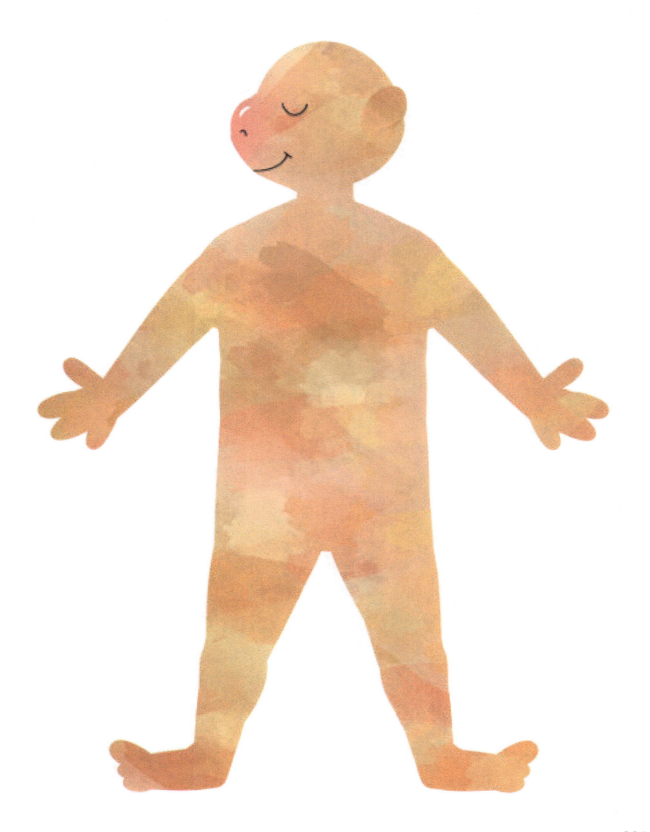

© Natalie Duhon

Point to the following body parts: brain, heart, lungs, stomach. Do you remember how these parts of our body are affected by our emotions? Take some time to review what you learned about the relationship between our physical and mental health.

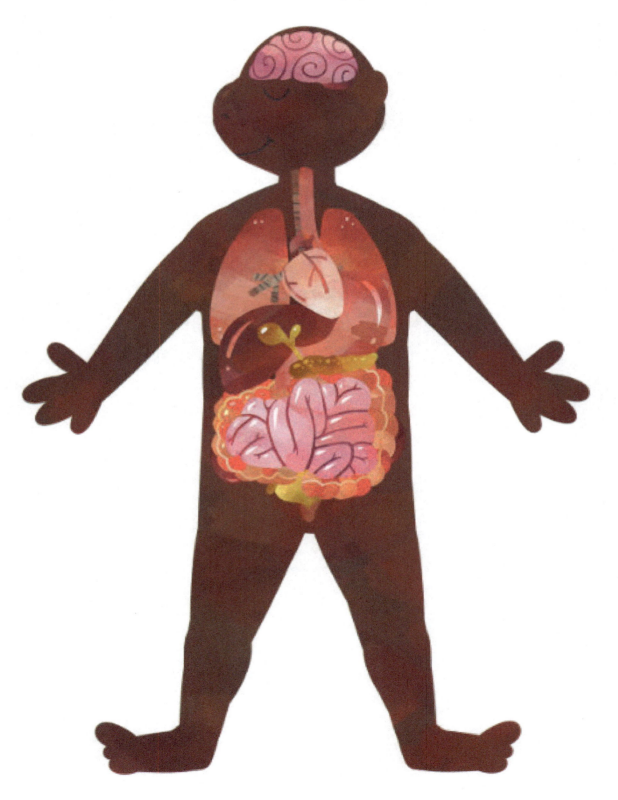

Animal Memory Match

Cut out and laminate the following cards. Play a game of memory match to improve your focus. Have fun and notice how this game can improve your mental health!

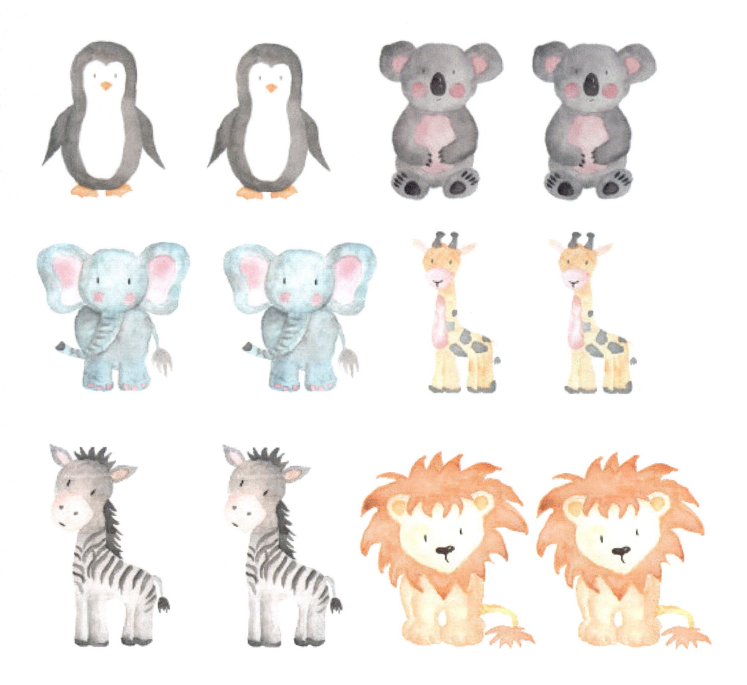

Intentionally left blank for double sided printing

Animal Memory Match (cont.)

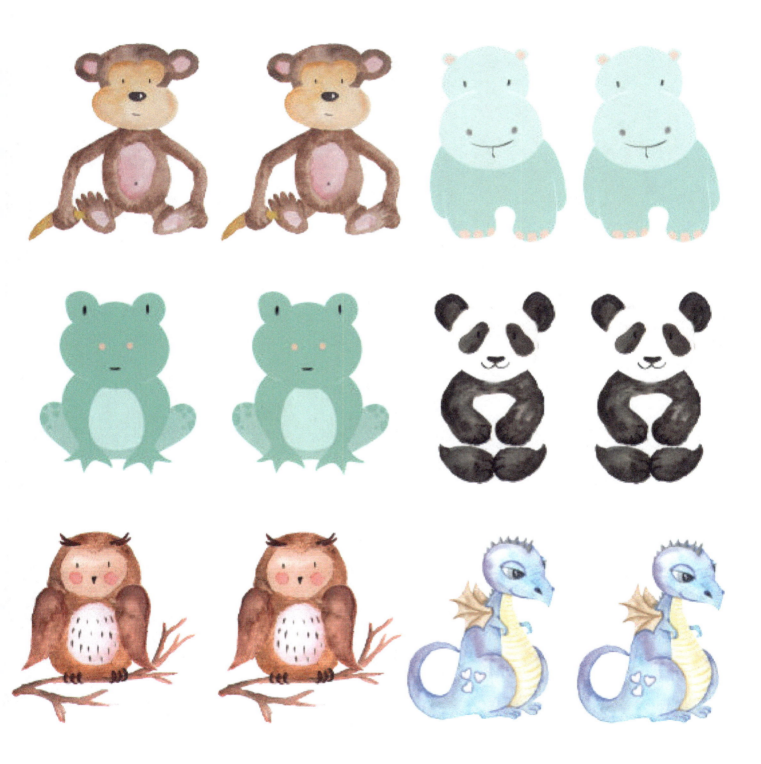

Intentionally left blank for double sided printing

Animal Memory Match

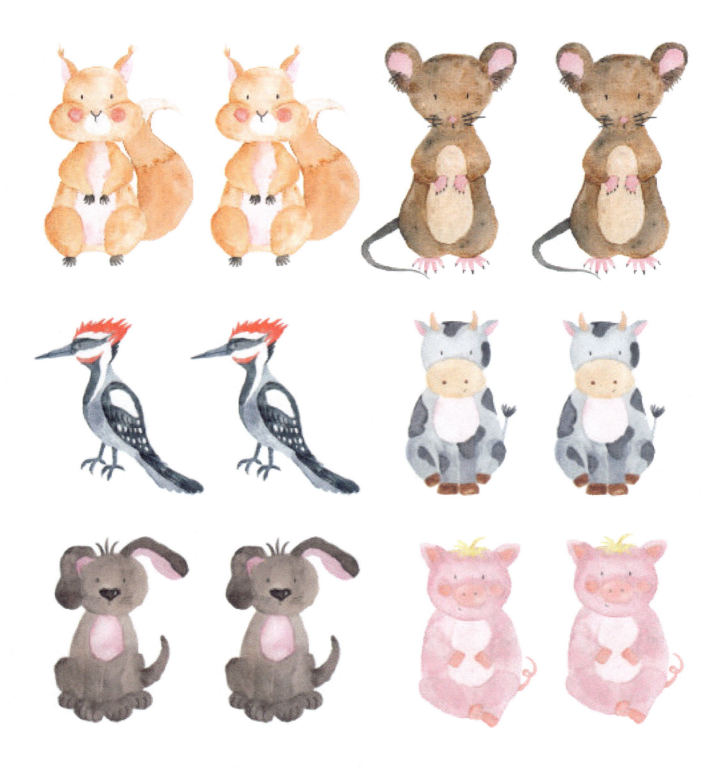

Intentionally left blank for double sided printing

BINGO Cards

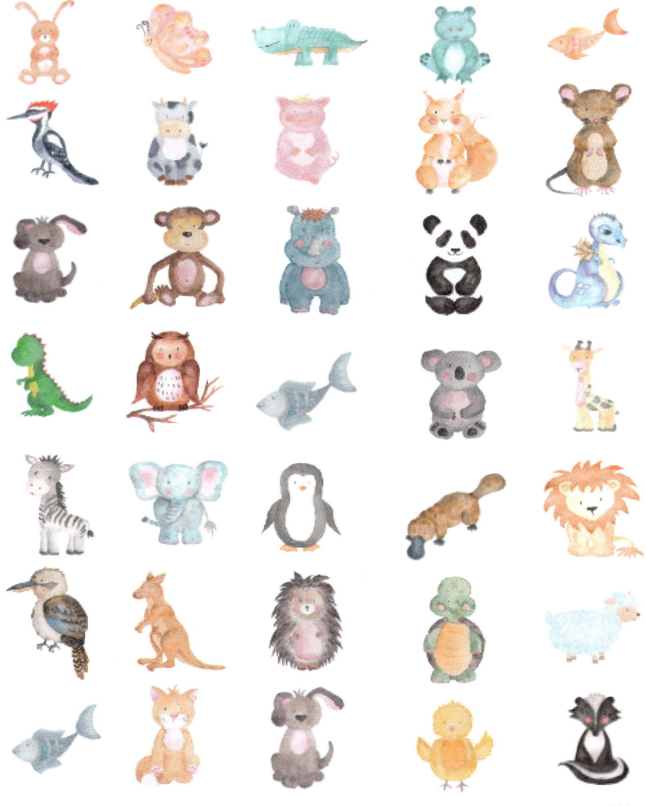

Intentionally left blank for double sided printing

Unscramble the emotion words.

dsa   _____

lgda   _____

dma   _____

pypah _____

rdsace _____

jyo   _____

voel   _____

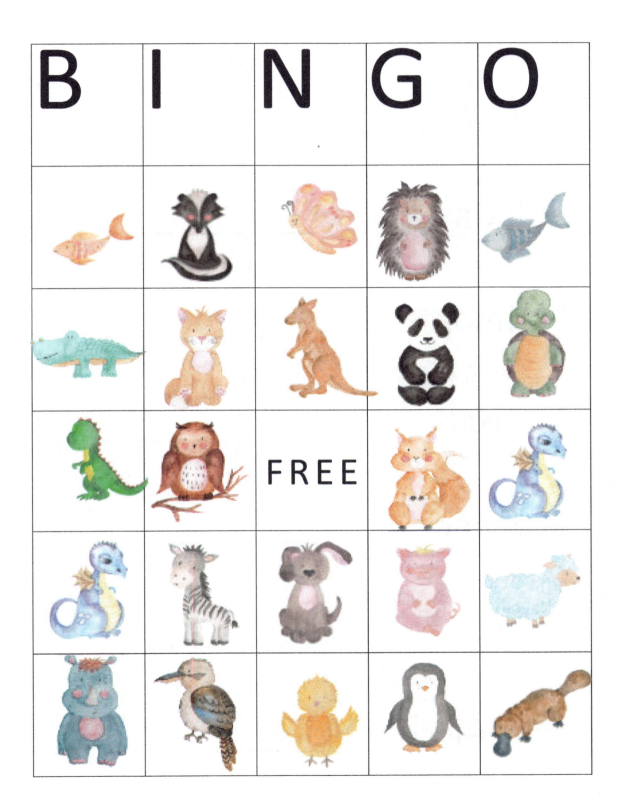

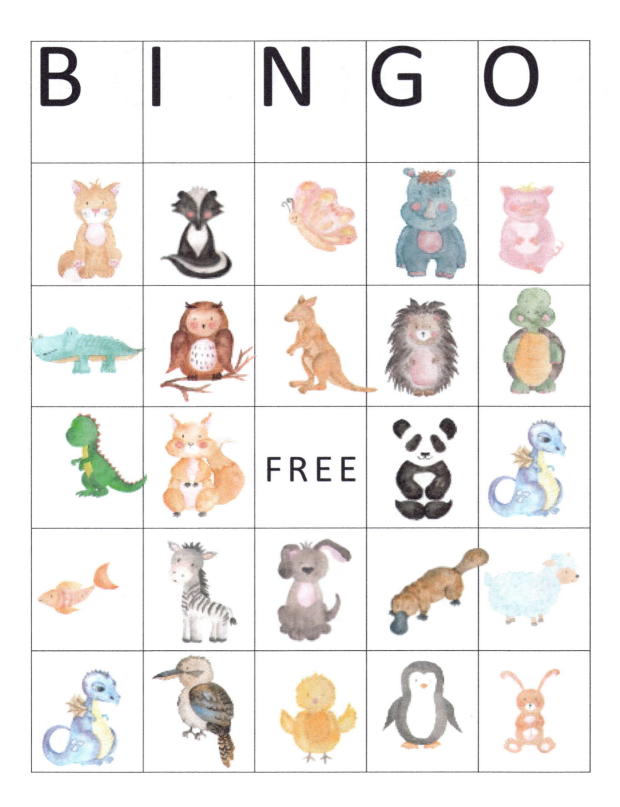

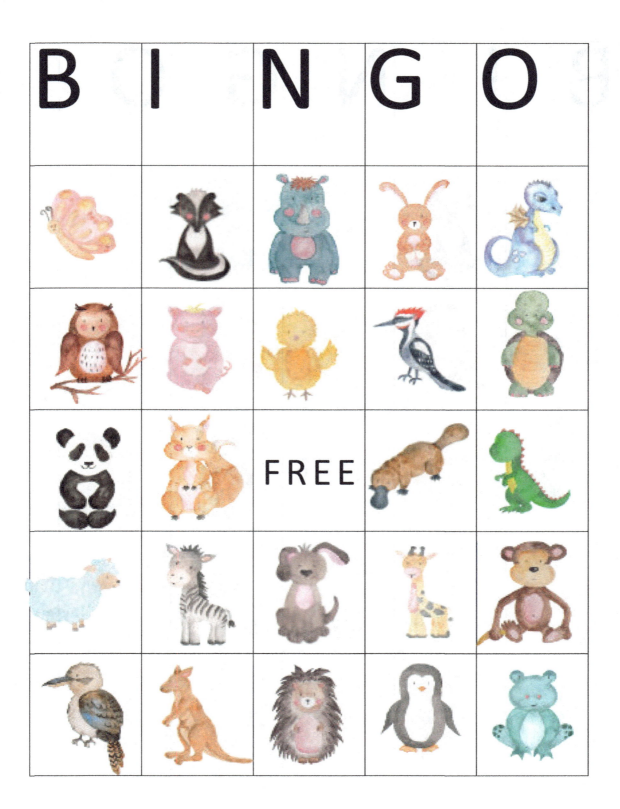

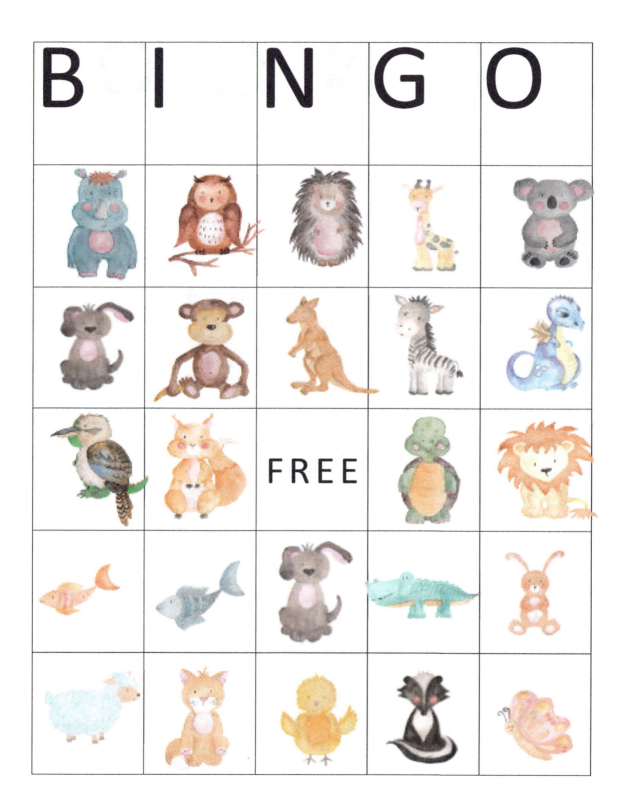

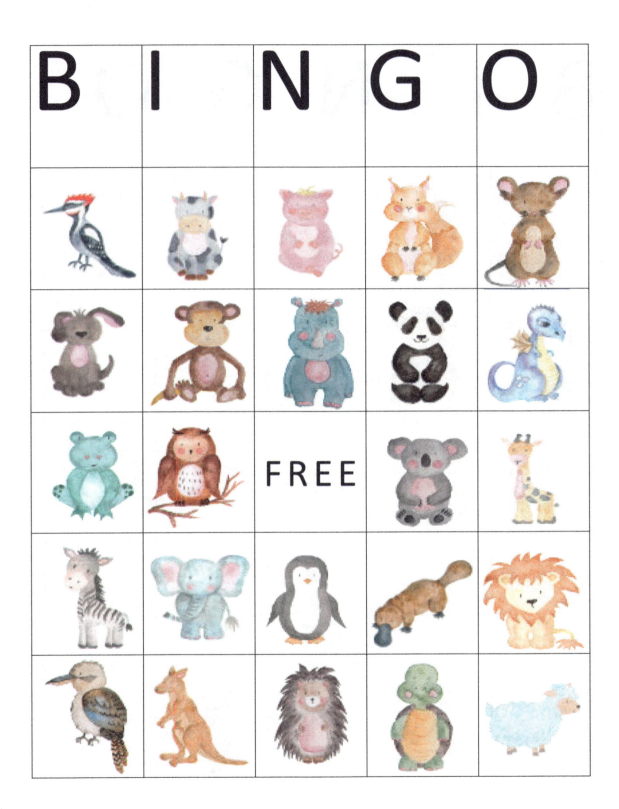

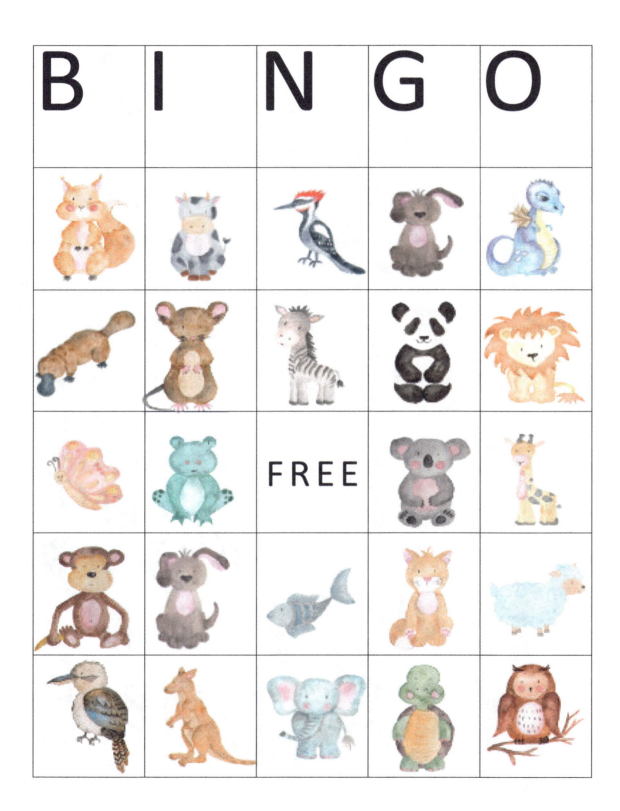

Print and laminate the following Bible posters to display in your homeschool room.

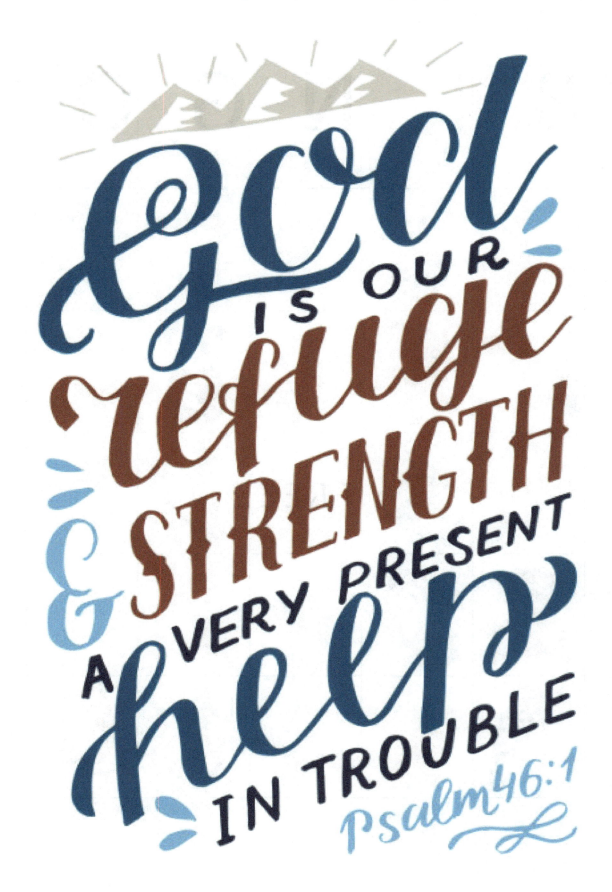

© Natalie Duhon

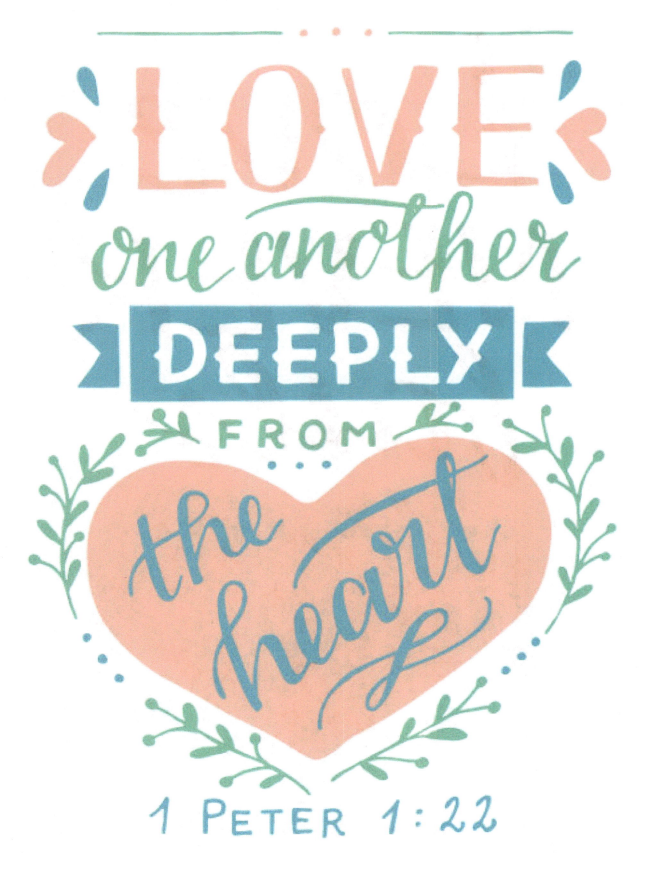

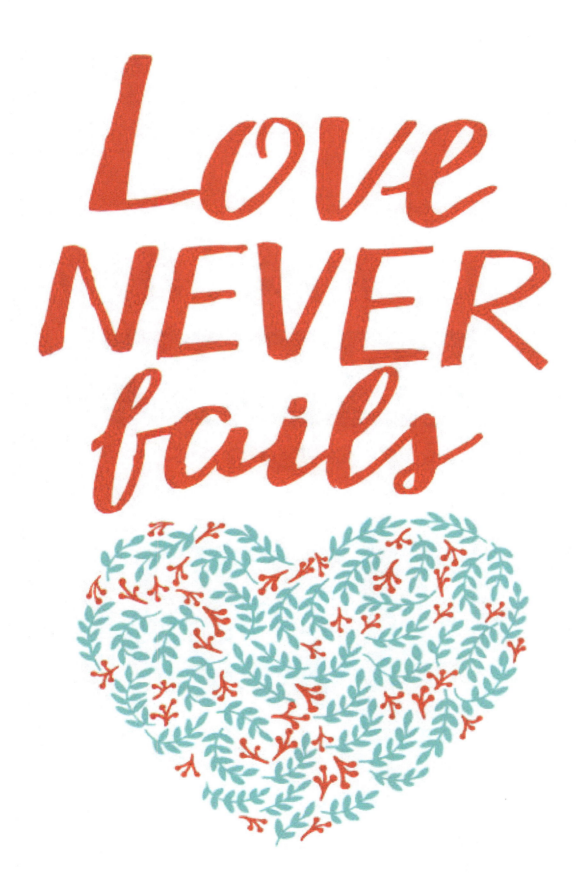

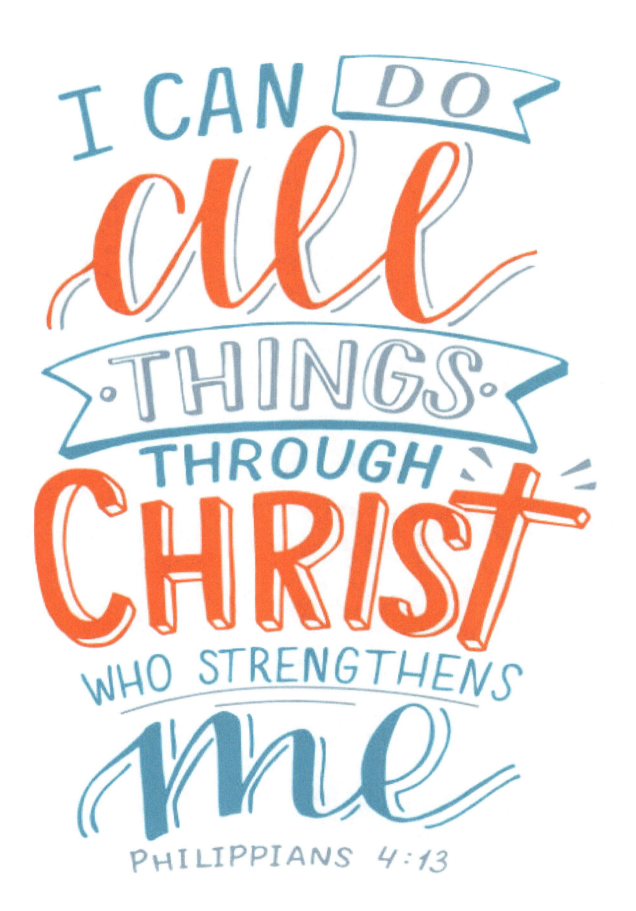

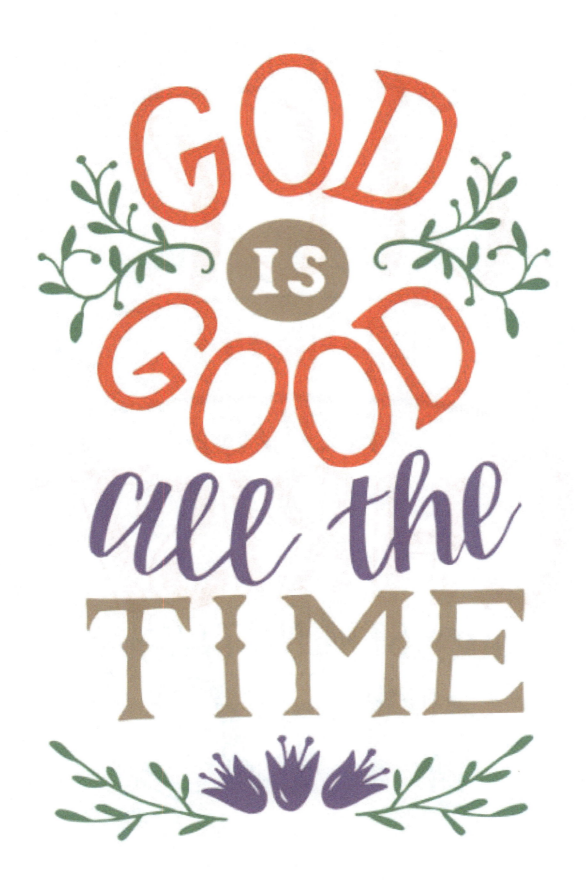

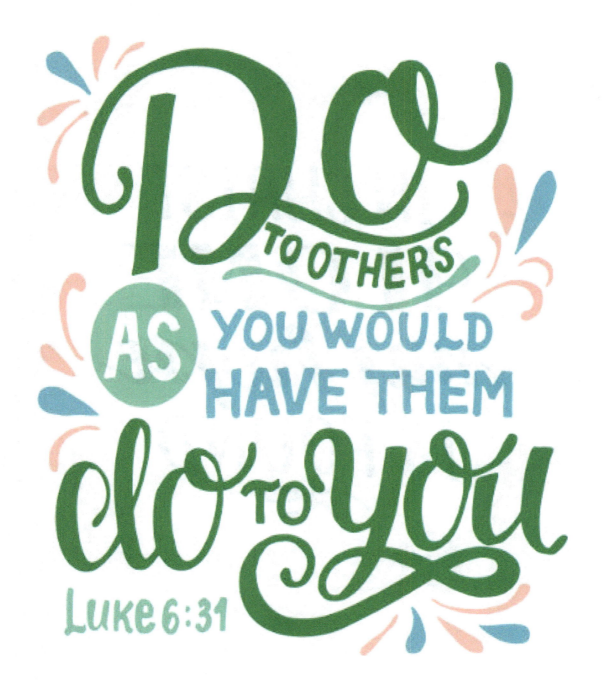

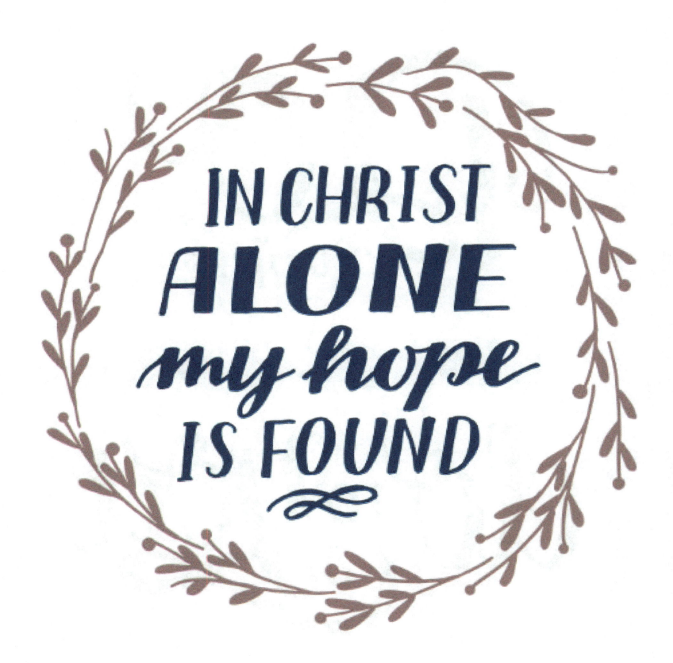

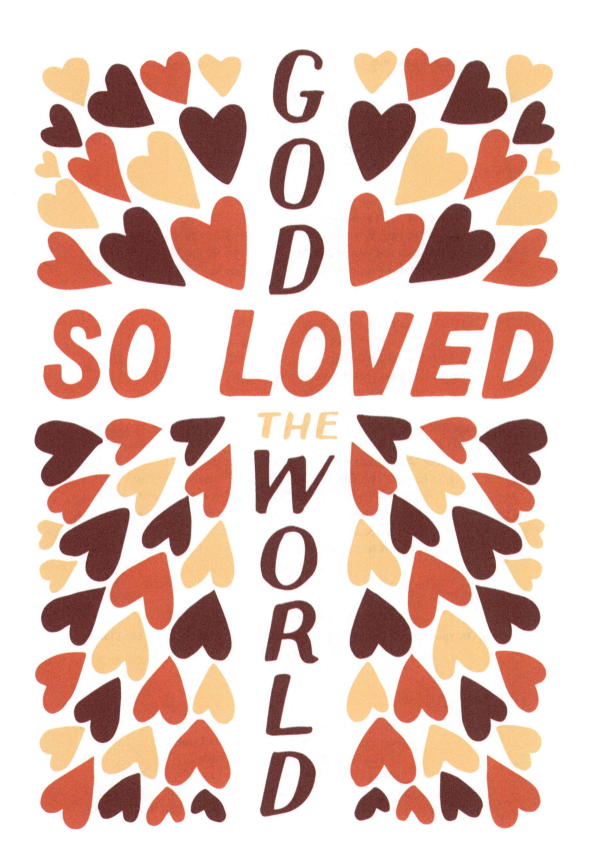

Recommend Reading (for children)

<u>Thoughts</u>
Captain Snout and the Super Power Questions by Daniel G. Amen, M.D.

<u>Emotions</u>
Kindness Is Cooler, Mrs. Ruler by Margery Cuyler
My Mouth is a Volcano! by Julia Cook
Wemberly Worried by Kevin Henkes
How Do YOU Feel? by Anthony Brown
The Way I Feel by Janan Cain
How Big Is Your Brave? by Ruth Soukup
What Am I Feeling? By Dr. Josh and Christi Straub
What Do I Do With Worry? by Dr. Josh and Christi Straub
God Cares When I'm Afraid by Stormie Omartian
Keeping Your Cool: A Book About Anger by Carolyn Larsen
Love Is Kind by Laura Sassi
Daniel Tiger's Thank You Day by Farrah McDoogle
Where'd My Giggle Go? by Max Lucado
I Am a Rainbow by Dolly Parton
God, I Need to Talk to You About My Bad Temper by Dan Carr
Don't Let Your Heart Feel Funny by Jerry and Kitty Thomas
In My Heart: A Book of Feelings by Jo Witek
Daniel Feels Left Out by Maggie Testa
The Feelings Book: The Care & Keeping of Your Emotions by Dr. Lynda Madison
I Am Human: A Book About Empathy by Susan Verde
A Children's Book About Emotions: Handling Your Ups and Downs by Joy Wilt
How to Take the Grrrr Out of Anger by Elizabeth Verdick
My Book of Feelings: A Book to Help Children with Attachment Difficulties, Learning or Developmental Disabilities Understand Their Emotions by Tracey Ross, Rosy Salaman
Visiting Feelings by Lauren Rubenstein
Keep Calm! My Stress-Busting Tips by Gina Bellisario
Thankful by Eileen Spinelli
The Great Big Book of Feelings by Mary Hoffman
Who Feels Scared? By Sue Graves
The Thankful Book by Todd Parr
How Do You Doodle? Drawing My Feelings and Emotions by Elise Gravel
ABC of Feelings by Bonnie Lui
The Hundred Dresses by Eleanor Estes

<u>Social Skills</u>
Tease Monster by Julia Cook
Making Friends is an Art! by Julia Cook
That's (not) Mine by Anna Kang
We Are (not) Friends by Anna Kang
Being Nice to Others: A Book About Rudeness by Carolyn Larsen
The Berenstain Bears Play a Fair Game by Stan and Jan Berenstain
Hands Are Not for Hitting by Martine Agassi

© Natalie Duhon

God, I Need to Talk to You About Hurting Others by Dan Carr
God, I Need to Talk to You About Disrespect by Susan Leigh
God, I Need to Talk to You About Bad Manners by Susan Leigh
God, I Need to Talk to You About Bad Words by Susan Leigh
God, I Need to Talk to You About Whining by Susan Leigh
God, I Need to Talk to You About Sharing by Dan Carr
The Berenstain Bears Get In a Fight by Stan and Jan Berenstain
Winnie the Pooh Friendship Day by Nancy Parent
Daniel Learns to Share by Becky Friedman
The Berenstain Bears and the Golden Rule by Stan and Jan Berenstain
Llama Llama and the Bully Goal by Anna Dewdney
The Berenstain Bears love Their Neighbors by Jan and Mike Berenstain
Join In and Play by Cheri Meiners
Calm-Down Time by Elizabeth Verdick
Teamwork Isn't My Thing, and I Don't Like to Share! By Julia Cook

Self-esteem
The Work of Your Hand by Jennifer Hall Rivera, EdD
Moo-Moo, I love You! by Tom Lichtenheld
Only You Can Be You! by Nathan and Sally Clarkson
You are Extraordinary by Craig and Samantha Johnson
One Big Heart by Linsey Davis
The Wonder That Is You by Glenys Nellis
I Love You This Much by Lynn Hodges and Sue Buchanan

Boundaries
Boundaries by Cornelia Spelman
Let's Talk About Body Boundaries, Consent, and Respect by Jayneen Sanders
Consent (For Kids): Boundaries, Respect, and Being in Charge of YOU by Rachel Brian

Other
Telling the Truth: A Book About Lying by Carolyn Larsen
God, I Need to Talk to You About Talking Back by Susan Leigh
God, I Need to Talk to You About Paying Attention by Dan Carr
God, I Need to Talk to You About Lying by Dan Carr
On Mission magazine by Gentle Classical Press

Recommended Resources (for children)
https://www.teacherspayteachers.com/Store/Natalie-Duhon
Emotiblocks by Miniland Educational
Little Folk Visuals pre-cut emotions
Emoji Cubes by Learning Resources
Emotion-OES by Carson Dellosa Education Store
Feelings Flips by Junior Learning
Let's Talk Cubes by Learning Resources
In the Season of Valentine's Day by Campfire Curriculums

© Natalie Duhon

<u>Recommended Reading</u> (for parents/caregivers)
Labels by Derek Griffon
Drawing Calm: Relax, Refresh, Refocus by Susan Evenson
Her Children Arise by Casey Hilty
Winning the War In Your Mind: Change Your Thinking, Change Your Life by Craig Groeschel
The Grave Robber by Mark Batterson
Mom Set Free by Jeannie Cunnion

<u>Recommended Resources</u> (for parents/caregivers)
Post Partum support: www.Psidirectory.com, www.Postpartum.net
Right Now Media
https://suicidepreventionlifeline.org/ (1-800-273-8255)
https://nami.org/Home
https://www.nimh.nih.gov/

REFERENCES

American Psychiatric Association: Diagnostic and Statistical Manual of Mental Disorders, Fifth Edition. Arlington, VA, American Psychiatric Association, 2013

Barlow, D. (2008). *Clinical Handbook of Psychological Disorders: A Step-by-Step Treatment Manual*. The Guilford Press.

Bauer, M., Kilbourne, A., Greenwald, D., Ludman, E. *Overcoming Bipolar Disorder: A Comprehensive Workbook for Managing Your Symptoms & Achieving Your Goals.* New Harbinger Publications, Inc.

Beck, J. (1995). *Cognitive Therapy: Basics and Beyond.* The Guilford Press.

Bellack, A., Mueser, K., Gingerich, S., Agresta, J. (2004). *Social Skills Training for Schizophrenia*. The Guilford Press.

Bernstein, J. (2017). *Mindfulness for Teen Worry: Quick & Easy Strategies to Let Go of Anxiety, Worry, & Stress.* Instant Help Books.

Bourne, E. (2020). *The Anxiety & Phobia Workbook* 7th edition. New Harbinger Publications, Inc.

Butler, G., Fennell, M., & Hackmann, A. (2010). *Cognitive-Behavioral Therapy for Anxiety Disorders: Mastering Clinical Challenges*. The Guilford Press

Burnes, D. (1999). *The Feeling Good Handbook*. Penguin Group

Centre for Clinical Interventions. (https://www.cci.health.wa.gov.au/Resources/For-Clinicians (2021)).

GetSelfHelp (2022). (https://getselfhelp.co.uk/problems/)

Johnson, S. (2004). *Therapist's Guide to Clinical Intervention: The 1-2-3's of Treatment Planning*. Second Edition. Academic Press

Johnsma, A. & Peterson, L. (2006). *The Complete Adult Psychotherapy Treatment Planner.* John Wiley & Sons, INC.

Lerner, H. (2005). *The Dance of Anger*. HarperCollins Publishers Inc.

McKay, M., Davis, M., & Fanning, P. (2011). *Thoughts & Feelings: Taking Control of Your Moods and Your Life.* Fourth Edition. New Harbinger Publications, Inc.

National Alliance on Mental Illness. (https://www.nami.org/About-Mental-Illness)

National Institute of Mental Health. (https://www.nimh.nih.gov/health/topics)

Perkinson, R. (2012). *Chemical Dependency Counseling: A Practical Guide.* SAGE Publications.

Shapiro, L. (2017). *The Panic Attack Workbook.* Between Sessions Resources.

Shapiro, L. (2017). *Overcoming Depression: 44 Therapeutic Activities to Bring Happiness and Fulfillment Back Into Your Life.* Between Sessions Resources.

Snowden, S. (2018). *Anger Management Workbook for Kids*. Althea Press.

Spradlin, S. (2003). *Don't Let Your Emotions Run Your Life*. New Harbinger Publications Inc.

Swarbrick, P. & Yudof, J. (2015). *Wellness in Eight Dimensions*. Collaborative Support Programs of NH, Inc.

Therapist Aid. (2022). https://www.therapistaid.com/

Thompson, R. (2003). *Counseling Techniques* Second Edition. Routledge Taylor & Francis Group.

Merriam-Webster, Incorporated. (2022). (https://www.merriam-webster.com/dictionary/emotion)

Image Credits

Cover and feelings faces (confident, confused, embarrassed, happy, joyful, mad, sad, scared, silly, surprised, thankful, worried) © Lauren Sibley Brasseaux

All other images purchased from Creative Market and are licensed for commercial use.

©https://creativemarket.com/juliabrnv/2281951-16300

©https://creativemarket.com/CreativequbeDesign/2750647

©https://creativemarket.com/Natdzho/6248246-THERAPY

©https://creativemarket.com/DigitalArtsi/1584922

©https://creativemarket.com/tanya.kart/2309473

©https://creativemarket.com/AlesyaPytskaya/6082789

©https://creativemarket.com/juliabrnv/6117521-8064

©https://creativemarket.com/OlliArtDesign/6520300

©https://creativemarket.com/paulaparaula/2485720

©https://creativemarket.com/ElenaDorosh/5837945

©https://creativemarket.com/FloraAndBear/5880088

©https://creativemarket.com/Ola-la-la/4699351

©https://creativemarket.com/Ylivdesign/3694785-100

©https://creativemarket.com/lana_elanor/4254271

©https://creativemarket.com/TopVectors/6109474

©https://creativemarket.com/writelovely/3084491

About the Author

Natalie DeMoor Duhon is a Licensed Professional Counselor in the state of Louisiana. She earned a Master of Science in Counselor Education and a Bachelor of Science in Child and Family Studies at the University of Louisiana at Lafayette. She resides in Lafayette, Louisiana with her husband and seven year old daughter. She has worked in the mental health field for over ten years. She has experience providing group and individual therapy in inpatient and outpatient settings. Natalie has homeschooled her daughter since preschool and her daughter is the inspiration for this curriculum.

Made in the USA
Coppell, TX
17 October 2023